The Woof and Warp

of Canine Pain

Treating Dogs with TCM

Second Edition

The Woof and Warp of Canine Pain
Treating Dogs with TCM
Second Edition

Second Edition Published in 2013 by
Planet Calamari Publishing
Alexandria, VA

First Edition Published in 2010

Cover created by Norman Kraft.

Typeset in LaTeX with the Bookman font.

Karma is real - don't steal.

Caution

This book is intended for practitioners of Chinese medicine who have been trained in Chinese herbal medicine and prescriptions, as well as TCM diagnosis and differentiation of disease. While this book may be useful to practitioners of other healing arts, canine acupuncture and Chinese herbal medicine are complex subjects, may present risks, and may be subject to state and local laws. Cases should be referred to a qualified practitioner of canine acupuncture and Chinese medicine.

The authors do not advocate nor endorse the use of Chinese medicine on animals by laypersons. Chinese medicine is a professional medicine. Laypersons interested in applying the treatments as described in this book to their dog or other animal should seek out a qualified professional practitioner of canine acupuncture and Chinese medicine.

To all suffering dogs.

Acknowledgments

I am grateful to my doggie soul mate, Merlin Mossa, a German Shepherd dog who was the inspiration and catalyst to begin a veterinary acupuncture practice. Not a day goes by that I do not think of him. Together with Nina and Liberty, these shepherds were the original Four Paws Acupuncture pack who taught me how to speak canine.

I am blessed to be married to a man of infinite patience and talent. I could not have done this class or book with out the help of my husband, Norman Kraft, L.Ac. My Love, thank you for your editing, recording, left brain skills and your sense of humor through all of it.

I thank my teachers at Pacific College of Oriental Medicine for your wisdom, knowledge and patience. And to the dear friends I made at PCOM, thank you for your sense of humor!

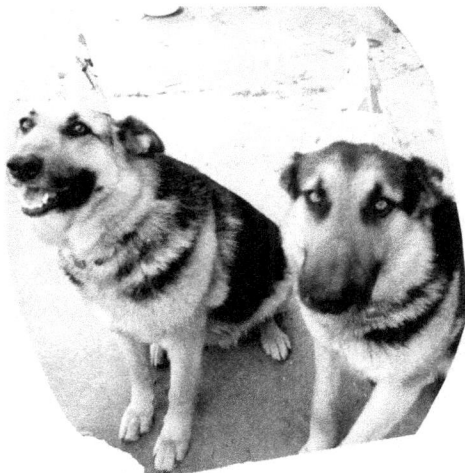

Contents

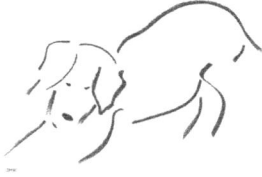

"Dogs are not our whole life,
but they make our lives whole."

Roger Caras

Introduction

The idea for this book has been nagging at me for several years. I tried to write this book with the idea of what I would say to someone who was just starting to treat dogs. Some of the things in this book are not from Traditional Chinese Medicine (TCM), however without some of these tips it is difficult to actually practice effective Chinese medicine on your dog patient.

Ted Kaptchuk's *The Web That Has No Weaver: Understanding Chinese Medicine* is required reading for most acupuncture students. Kaptchuk makes writing an art of painting words to explain the most obscure concepts of Chinese Medicine. It was one of the books that actually made sense that confusing first year of acupuncture school, and the book still inspires me.

The first time I heard the terms Woof and Warp (the title of a chapter in *The Web The Has No Weaver*), was in a class discussing Kaptchuk's theories. These terms come from weaving, where the woof is the thread going one way and the warp is the threads that weave across it. The term has come to mean the underlying structure of something. Treating dogs with Traditonal Chinese Medicine is not just about diagnosis the way we were taught it in school. It is a dance. Its a puzzle. How can we take the pieces of knowledge we learned and treat our canine patients who do not speak the same language as we do? How can we think like a dog? What can we learn? How can we weave our skills as a practitioner while thinking like a dog.

While I was attending PCOM San Diego, I had a 12 year old German Shepherd named Merlin. He was my dog soul mate. During this time he was diagnosed with arthritis and hip dysplasia. The vet wanted to "put him down." Instead I fired the vet and learned how to treat Merlin with acupuncture, herbs, and a new diet. He lived to be almost 15, fully three years longer than anyone expected.

Thus began my obsession with treating dogs with TCM and learning as much as possible about dogs, their ailments, nature, hereditary factors and behavior.

This book is an overview of methods for treating canine

pain and *Bi* syndromes with Chinese herbal medicine, acupuncture, nutrition, supplements and lifestyle changes. It also contains tips on how to actually think outside the box and think like a dog. First tip: Learn to say these two mantras over and over: "Good Boy!" or "Good Girl!" and "Do you want a cookie?"

This book is geared toward licensed acupuncturists with significant herbal training, a sense of humor and a love of dogs.

Introduction to the Second Edition

It has been almost five years since I first began writing The Woof & Warp of Canine Pain, Treating Dogs with TCM. That's 35 dog years. In that time, a lot has changed. There has been an increasing awareness of problems in the the dog food industry, with public recalls of so many pet foods. The pet industry, under the microscope of the general public (and the Internet) was forced to deal with issues that were previously swept under the rug.

Acupuncture is no longer considered as *wooie wooie* as it once was. Holistic veterinary care is now accepted by many veterinarians. Unfortunately many state laws still prohibit licensed acupuncturists with extensive training to treat animals, while allowing veterinarians with only a few weekends of classes to do so. I personally stood before the Massachusetts Veterinary Board in 2010 to defend my right to treat animals with acupuncture — and won. I encourage others (who have nerves of steel) to do the same.

On a happier note, we adopted a rescue dog from the SPCA of Tennessee in 2010. Quan Yin is a mix of Border Collie, Newfoundland and Dragon. Filled with love and a variety of quirks from her adventures of being abandoned in the floods of 2010. Because of her, I am grateful to have learned a few more modalities and remedies to add to my repertoire for treating dogs. As always "think outside the box" has been my motto when treating animals. Just like humans, all animals have a distinct personality. No two behave the same, and their bodies don't react to remedies in the same way. And not all remedies are created equal.

In this second edition I have added more information on Bach Flower Essences, healthy and therapeutic cooking recipes for dogs, and a few products that I recommend to help calm dogs and cats.

In Dog We Trust,

jeanie mossa kraft, L.Ac.

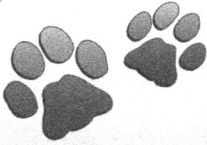

August 16th is the
feast day of St Roch,
the patron saint of dogs.

Chapter 1

The Practice of Canine Acupuncture

Needless to say it is important to be a "dog person" if you intend to treat dogs. Remember, too, that each dog has their own personality. A very wise veterinarian once told me that he treats all of his patients like they are little people. While dogs are not people, they have the same basic needs that humans do. Treat them with compassion and respect, and arm yourself with a few healthy treats or a ball to be on the safe side! You may need to think outside the box for a treatment plan for some of your dog patients. What you learned in acupuncture school needs to be adapted to canines.

Finally, be prepared to be covered in fur, drool and dog cookie crumbs!

When treating dogs you have to also remember that you will dealing with the owner as well. Sometimes you will find that the dog is more cooperative than the owner during the session.

The first session I go over everything that may help the dog's condition during the initial intake (discussed later). If there needs to be a change in diet or supplements added I give the owner a list of what I recommend and where they can find it. I personally do not sell anything. I find people are more compliant if they do not think you are recommending products to make extra income.

During housecall sessions, I have had owners cooking dinner, heard screaming matches on the phone, watched them yell at their kids, text their family and friends, surf the Internet, and watch TV. One actually left the room to take a bath. I have been hit with a broom by a 3 year old. Whacked on the head with a Tonka truck by her brother, asked if I would take out the garbage and told what points I should needle by someone who had never experienced acupuncture. This is a reality of housecalls, but these noisy and distracting activities are not helpful to the dog's treatment. I now try to minimize these distractions, by educating the owners to become partners in helping to create a quieter, healing environment.

Most dog owners mean well. However since you are the health care provider you need to set the boundaries for the treatment session as well as educate the owner on their responsibilities for caring for a sick dog before the appointment.

Owners need to be advised that acupuncture is not a cure all. Don't assume that they are aware of the cumulative effect of acupuncture. In most cases, a course of treatment will require at least 3-6 sessions for noticeable results. One session is a waste of time and money.

The owner must also be counseled to feed the dog a healthy diet, clean water, give adequate exercise, and to continue with medication if prescribed by their veterinarian. If you prescribe herbs you need to instruct the owner how often and how much to give the dog, as well as methods of administration. You may want to send a followup email with a reminder of what you discussed.

If the dog is living in a house with hard tile or hardwood floor you may need to suggest throw rugs or runners down the stairs. You are the spokesperson for the dog, who is counting on you to communicate on their behalf.

Here are a few guidelines that may help you more effectively educate owners to help create a more relaxing session for the dog. I make sure the owner is aware of these guidelines before I schedule the first session. This avoids uncomfortable situations later. I also send an email with my request and guidelines for a relaxing house call.

- The owner must be present in the room the entire session. He or she must also be fully attentive and not doing distracting things such as talking on the phone, texting, putting dishes away, cooking, etc. This is important – a present owner may be the difference between an effective treatment and getting bit.
- Schedule the session when the household is quiet and there will be fewer disturbances. Poor times include when children are just getting home from school or the owner is having furniture delivered and similar chaotic parts of the day.

- All TV, radio and music must be off while I am there, unless the music is relaxing and helpful toward relaxing the dog. It is in the best interest of the dog to have quiet and the owner's full attention.
- No smoking while I am in the home. Dogs don't like smoking, no matter what the owner says.
- If there are children in the home they must not be allowed to disturb the dog during treatment. They are welcome to watch quietly.

The owner must be cooperative partners in their dog's health. If they are not willing to put my recommendations to use, such as changing diet or daily massage with liniment, they are compromising the effectiveness of the treatments. If the owner is not willing to do these things, I may tell them flat out that they are wasting their money and my time.

Also, expect the unexpected. You never know when the dog is just going to stand up and shake all the needles out or have to go to the bathroom just as the treatment is started. Canine acupuncture requires a sense of humor.

As an acupuncturist I feel I must defend our profession.

Nothing makes me crazier than to hear that acupuncture does not work from an owner who has only had one session and feeds the dog Alpo!

Finally, be polite and professional. You are a representative to our profession, and you are doing your work in someone's home.

It is very helpful to call your clients to see how the dog did after the first session. Be available for questions or concerns. Give your clients printed information whenever possible. The more informed the client is the more they will help you.

If you are one of those acupuncturist who is treating dogs in a clinic, most of these guidelines apply. You have an opportunity to create an effective healing space, and you should put as much effort into that as you would for a human patient.

Please note if you treat humans too, in most states it is illegal and unethical for you to treat your dog patients in the same treatment space as your human patients. Many people are allergic to dogs, and dogs can also bring ticks and fleas into your clinic.

1.1 Know Your Dog Breeds

Numerous national kennel clubs have assigned breeds to groups based on the purpose for which they were originally bred and developed. Some breed characteristics are common across groups and many hereditary factors are common in certain groups, and tend toward common health problems. Below, are listed some common breed categories and the health challenges common to them.

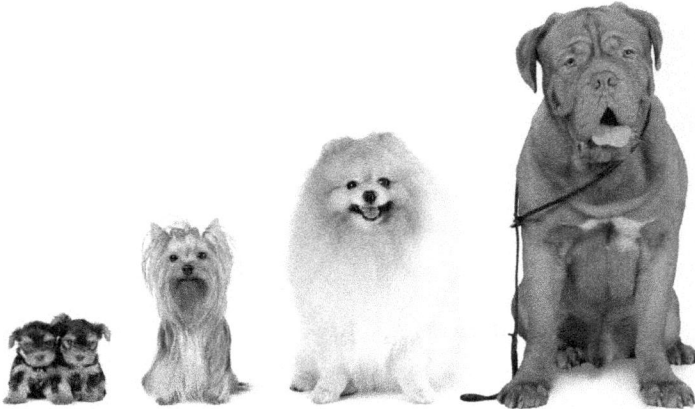

Please note that there are too many breed categories to list here. A breed neither protects nor causes any disease or disorder. However some breeds tend to present with certain illnesses. For example the larger breeds are prone to skeletal disorders because of the size of their skeleton. It has been said "The bigger the dog, the bigger the vet bill!"

Sporting Dog Group

The Sporting Dog group includes pointers, setters, retrievers and many spaniels. The most common are the Labrador Retriever and the Golden Retriever. These dogs are active dogs and love to run and swim. They were developed to aid hunters by searching, flushing out and retrieving game. Because of this, these dogs are obsessed with having something in their mouths such as a ball, stick and especially food! These dogs are usually good natured and can be bribed with treats to behave during an acupuncture session.

Sporting dogs are prone to knee problems, hip and elbow dysplasia, intestinal disorders, cancer, and cardiac problems.

Working Dog Group

These are the dogs that love to have jobs. They need a purpose or a job to be satisfied. They make excellent guard dogs. This group includes breeds such as the

Rottweiler, Doberman Pinscher, Akita, Alaskan Malamute, Samoyed, Siberian Husky, Great Pyrenees, and Newfoundland. These dogs are very intelligent and are very protective of their surroundings and owners. Treat these dogs with respect.

Working dogs are big and are prone to arthritis, elbow or hip dysplasia, bloat, wobblers, and various neurological disorders.

Toy Dog Group

These are the very small and miniature dog breeds, including the Yorkshire Terriers, Toy Poodles, Shih Tzus, Pugs, Pomeranians and Maltese. Toy dog breeds are very difficult to housebreak and the smaller the dog the more difficult is to train them. Unfortunately some of these dogs will urinate in the house if the owner does not train them at a young age. I have found they are the most difficult of all the dog groups to treat with acupuncture. They are wiry and have a very nervous energy. It is difficult to convince the dog to allow the needles to stay in for more than 5 minutes. I usually use the laser on these breeds.

Smaller dogs seem to be more prone to eye and skin

disorders, allergies, respiratory disorders, and Heart Fire.

Terrier Group

This group includes breeds that were developed in Great Britain to hunt small animals. These fiesty dog breeds have been domesticated but they are still fairly active and require training. They need stimulation. These are not dogs who should be left alone for several hours unattended (or else they may destroy what ever they can). The group includes the Airedale Terrier, Fox Terrier, Jack Russell Terrier and the Kerry Blue Terrier. Other popular terriers include the Yorkshire Terrier, Boston Terrier, Scottish Terrier and Cairn Terrier. These dogs are a challenge to treat. They are very smart and will watch your every move. They can also get very cranky. Do not force this dog to do anything he or she does not like or you may get bit!

Hound Group

These dog breeds have a great sense of smell. They can smell something that's practically in the next city.

They were developed to follow game either by sight or by smell. Sighthounds include the Afghans, Greyhounds, Salukis, Borzoi, and Irish Wolfhounds. They need exercise and love to run. Scent hounds include the Bloodhounds, Bassets, Beagles and all the other various hound dogs. These dogs are also very intelligent and will usually check you out by sniffing your clothing and anything you are carrying.

Herding Dog Groups

The dog breeds in this group were developed to herd and control cattle and sheep. They are considered to be some of the most intelligent breeds. This group includes the Shetland Sheepdog, Border Collie, Collie, German Shepherd, and Belgian Shepherd. They are one of my favorite groups of dogs to treat. Most seem to understand you are there to help them and will cooperate. They aim to please their owners and protect their domain. Most are very happy to be given a ball or a treat. And always praise these dogs when they are cooperating. Give them a "good boy!" or "good girl!" more often for a more effective session.

Unfortunately herding dogs suffer from several hereditary diseases such as hip or elblow dysplasia, knee problems, arthritis in old age, neurological disorders, and cancer and epilepsy.

Non-sporting Dog Group

These are the dog breeds that just don't seem to fit well in any other group. The breeds in this misfit group range from miniature dog breeds, like the Bichon Frise, to the larger Chow Chow, the Dalmatian, Bulldog and even the Boston Terrier.

Dalmations, in particular, are prone to intestinal problems, urinary disorders, deafness and arthritis.

1.2   Basic Canine Anatomy

Dogs have similar skeletal anatomy to humans. If you imagine a person in the yoga "Downward Dog" pose, you can visualize where most of the bones and joints would be on a dog. There are a few differences. For one, dogs basically walk on the balls of their feet, and the "heel" is above the ground. If you make sure to count your joints on the front and back legs, you'll be fine.

Also, there are minor differences in a dog's vertebral column. This can be a factor when counting vertebrae to locate UB points. Dogs have:

- 7 cervical vertebrae

- 13 thoracic vertebrae (where the 13 ribs are attached)

- 7 lumbar vertebrae

- 3 Sacral vertebrae

- 23 tail vertebrae

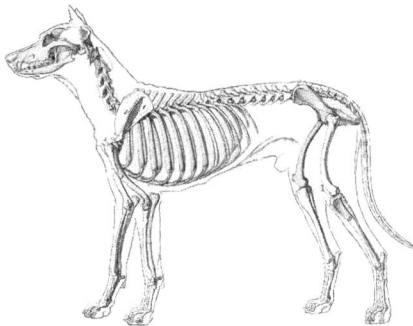

1.3 Taking a Canine Health History

As with your human patients, when treating a dog be advised to learn as much about him as you can before

working with him or her. This means taking a complete
veterinary history, including:

- Dog Name and age of dog
- Breed
- Purebred or mixed Breed?
- Is this a rescue dog?
- Name of Veterinarian and Phone Number
- Veterinarian's Diagnosis
- Full Medical History (including surgeries, shots, etc.)
- Symptoms (from the owner's point of view)
- Onset of symptoms (when did the problem begin?)
- What makes it worse? What makes it better?
- Is the dog panting abnormally?
- Is the dog crying or yelping on movement?
- Is the dog barking more than usual?
- Color and shape of the dog's tongue.
- Are the dog's bowel movements normal? Loose stool? Dry stool?
- Any bladder issues, urinary tract infections, and/or incontinence?
- Does the dog yelp or cry if touched? If so, where?
- Does the dog get exercise? How much?
- List of fears (thunder, fireworks, noise, etc)

- List of medications

- List of supplements

- Description of diet (including brand of food, table scraps, and treats)

- Are the symptoms worsened by cold or hot weather?

- Does the pain move around the body?

- Is the dog food-based or toy-based (prefers treats or a toy?)

- Where does the dog sleep? What is the dog's quality of sleep?

- Are there other animals in the same household? Do they get along? Who is the alpha?

- What is the dog allergic too?

- Does the dog have a history of biting?

1.4 Canine Diagnosis

You already know the signs and symptoms of Chinese syndromes in humans. These same syndromes also apply to dogs, and most diagnostic methods are the same. There is little or no pulse diagnosis with dogs, but tongue diagnosis is very useful as well as many of the diagnostic methods of looking, hearing, smelling and touching. A pale tongue is still a pale tongue, red eyes are still red eyes: trust your professional instincts in treating dogs.

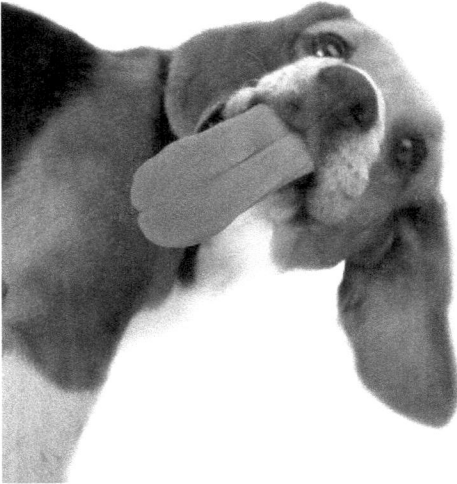

Tongue Diagnosis

The same principals apply to humans and dogs when it comes to tongue diagnosis. The only quirk in the system is that certain breeds have black or black spots on their tongue naturally. This should be taken into consideration when observing the tongue.

A difficulty in canine tongue diagnosis is trying to get the dog to show you its tongue. Sometimes I will offer a treat in hopes he will open his mouth. Another trick is to yawn in front of the dog. Usually they will yawn back. If all else fails, be watchful and eventually the dog will opens his or her mouth. **I do not recommended that you stick your hand or a tongue depressor in a dog's mouth.** That's how practitioners get bit.

A normal dog's tongue should have a thin white coat. Just like humans, if the coat is thick and white there may be cold and possibly dampness. A yellow coat means there is damp heat in the body. If the tongue is greasy then there may be phlegm.

A dry red shriveled tongue indicates yin deficiency and possibly Kidney deficiency. A purple tongue usually means liver blood stagnation. Pale tongue indicates blood deficiency.

Some dogs, like St Bernards, drool which may make it messy or difficult to see the coat of the tongue. Be patient. Unlike humans, with whom you get all your tongue information in one viewing, canine tongue diagnosis may come in parts. Also ask the owner if the dog just ate. This may effect the color or moisture on the tongue.

If you need to review tongue diagnosis I recommend reviewing *Tongue Diagnosis in Chinese Medicine* by Giovanni Maciocia. Even though the book covers human tongues, the same principals apply to dogs.

Pulse

In my experience, taking a dog's pulse is one of the most difficult aspects of diagnosing. It takes effort and skill, and the cooperation of the dog. Once again the same principals apply with human and dog pulse. In a perfect world you would attempt to take the dog's pulse on his wrists just as you would a human. It is very difficult to feel and some dogs will not allow you to touch their paws.

Another method is to palpate the femoral artery inside the back hind leg, very close to the dog's groin. Many dogs are not too thrilled about this method. According to Cheryl Schwartz, at the femoral artery, the first position is the pulse closest to the dog's groin and the third is the farthest away.

Personally I have not had much success taking dog's pulses. Even when one is felt it is hard to determine if my hand is in the correct spot for each organ.

To read more about this method I recommend reading *Four Paws, Five Directions* by Cheryl Schwartz, DVM.

Common Syndromes in Dogs

Some of the most common syndromes for dogs are combinations of Qi and Blood deficiency. Below is a review of these syndromes, with diagnostic markers as they apply to dogs:

Signs and Symptoms of Blood Deficiency

- Dry, brittle or patchy hair or nails
- Dry, red eyes (take into consideration dog breed - some naturally have red eyes. Other factors, such as allergies can also cause red eyes.)
- Dull eyes (Liver Blood)
- Pale, dry tongue with little or no coat
- Dry nose
- Pale nose
- Insomnia

Signs and Symptoms of Qi Deficiency

- Fatigue and/or easily tired
- Loose stools
- Diarrhea, gas, digestive problems
- Flabby tongue
- Pale tongue

- Shortness of breath
- Shallow panting
- Weak barking
- Worry

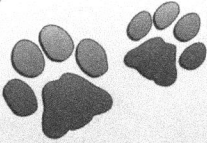

October 4th is the feast day of St Francis, patron saint of animals.

Chapter 2

Dogs and Pain

Dogs do talk, but they only speak canine. Since most people do not speak fluent canine, an ailment can go undetected until the dog begins to show signs of pain or begins to act out of character. Observation is a major part in diagnosing a dog. In the next section I will be discussing the signs and symptoms of pain and/or stress in dogs.

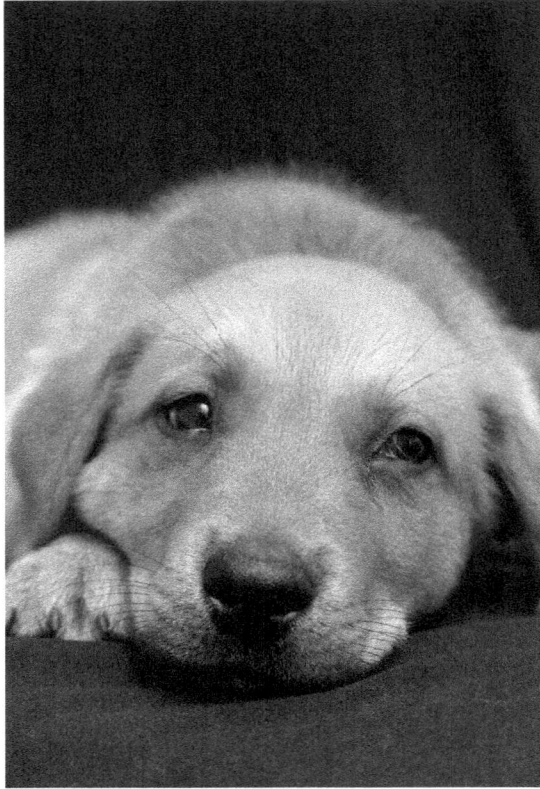

2.1   Causes of Pain

Unfortunately there are often times when the owner
cannot pinpoint how the pain began. Dogs may injure
themselves when there are no witnesses. Playing too
hard, over-doing a walk, falling off a couch or bed, being tossed about in the back seat of a car, and children
throwing toys are just some of the common causes of
pain and injury.

Here are a few more causes and symptoms of pain in dogs:

Causes:

- Injury
- Trauma
- Broken or fractured bones
- Sprains, contusions
- Herniated disc
- Arthritis
- Other disease
- Old age

Symptoms:

- Panting or crying due to pain
- Dog finds it difficult to get up after laying down
- Stiffness in legs
- Limping
- Hind leg stiffness
- Laying down during a walk
- Bunny hopping
- Difficulty walking on hardwood floors
- Symptoms worsened by cold damp or hot humid weather

2.2   Dogs and Stress

You wouldn't think a dog has much to be stressed about, but when they are experiencing pain and dysfunction, dogs can begin to show signs of stress and anxiety. They worry about whether they can walk down stairs safely, across hardwood floors without slipping. They worry that they don't jump as well, and may fall. They especially worry about food! Here are some of the causes and symptoms of stress in dogs:

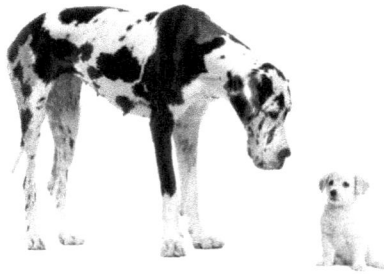

Causes of Stress in Dogs:

- Hunger
- Thirst
- Loud noises (thunder, fireworks, music)

- Clothing associated with pain, abuse or fear (e.g. baseball hats, gloves)
- Changing residence
- Pain or discomfort
- Vet visits
- Changes in domestic life
- New baby or other pet
- Owner's stress, fighting, arguments
- Meal time is missed

Symptoms of Stress in Dogs:

- Glazed eyes
- Weight loss
- Loss of appetite
- Hyperactivity
- Restless behavior
- Barking or whining for no apparent reason
- Extra naughty behavior

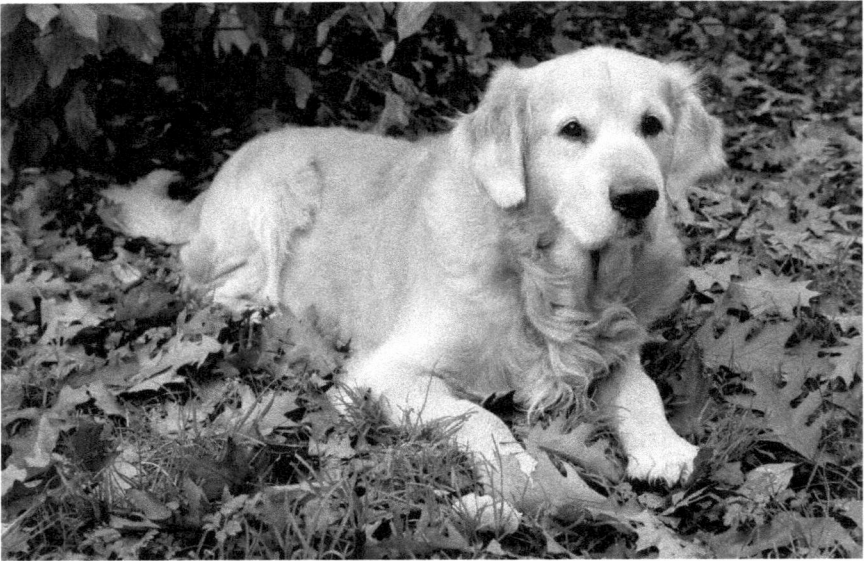

2.3   Arthritis

One of the most common causes of pain and stress in dogs is arthritis, particularly affecting older and larger dogs. In Chinese medicine arthritis is known as Bi Syndrome.

In western terms arthritis is one of the most common forms of pain and stress in dogs. Most older dogs suffer from some form of arthritis. Depending on the breed, age and size of dog the symptoms can vary from mild to the severe, joint deforming arthritis that we see in people.

Arthritis in Chinese medicine is called Bi Zheng, which translates as painful obstruction syndrome. The flow of Qi and Blood is blocked causing pain and joint movement limitations. Most commonly, these conditions are made worse by the Chinese pathogens Wind, Heat, Cold and Damp. Many dogs suffering from arthritis will show signs of pain during cold damp or hot humid weather.

Many older dogs have some form of bi syndrome. They often also suffer from Kidney Yin and or Yang deficiency, as well as Liver Blood Deficiency. Usually these dogs have a combination of these patterns, making diagnosis a complex process. Close examination of the signs and symptoms, as well as a good history from the owner are the keys to the proper diagnosis.

Dogs who have had bone injuries in the past are more prone to having arthritis when they get older.

Signs and Symptoms of Canine Arthritis

Many dog owners can not tell when their dog has arthritis since dogs can not tell them about their pain or symptoms. Usually it is not until the dog is in severe pain or symptoms actually appear that the owner takes the dog to the vet. Most vets will do X-rays to determine how far along the arthritis is.

Here are some of the signs and symptoms to look out for:

- Change in behavior
- Difficulty in getting up from the floor
- Stiffness while walking, trying to sit or lay
- Walking carefully
- Slowly walking
- No longer jumping
- Carefully walking up or down stairs
- Playing less
- Sleeping more

Treatment Strategies for Canine Arthritis

Acupuncture provides pain relief and increases mobility for most arthritic dogs. Given the cumulative effect of acupuncture over time, the first course of treatments should be acupuncture once per week for about 6 weeks. This is then followed by "tune-ups" every 2-4 weeks, as needed to continued relief.

2.4 Hip and Elbow Dysplasia

Hip dysplasia is also a very common cause of pain in older and larger dogs, with some overlap with arthritis in symptoms. Dysplasia occurs when the ball of the femur bone no longer fits tightly against the socket in the hip bone. This causes too much movement in the joint, and results in bone on bone wear and tear which causes pain. The dog will also eventually develop pain in its knees, back or elbows due to changes in body geometry. Though is it not arthritis, hip dysplasia may be seen as a type of bi syndrome: bony bi. The hereditary aspect of hip dysplasia implies Kidney Yin or Essence deficiency as well.

In Western medicine, Hip dysplasia is not the same thing as arthritis in the hips however it is one of the most common causes of arthritis in the hips.

Symptoms of Hip Dysplasia

Once again the dog cannot tell the owner he has hip dysplasia! Here are some of the signs and symptoms to look for:

- Difficulty getting up from the floor

- Decreased playing or activity
- Lameness in rear limbs
- Hesitation or refusal to go up stairs, jump or stand on hind legs
- Swaggering gait
- Pain in the hip area
- Sore after exercise

Elbow Dysplasia

Elbow dysplasia is a hereditary disease in which the elbow joints of the front legs are malformed. Symptoms of lameness will usually appear in the pup around 7 to 10 months of age. Western medicine treats it with anti-inflammatories and surgery. All breeds are susceptible to the disease but it is most common in the larger breeds.

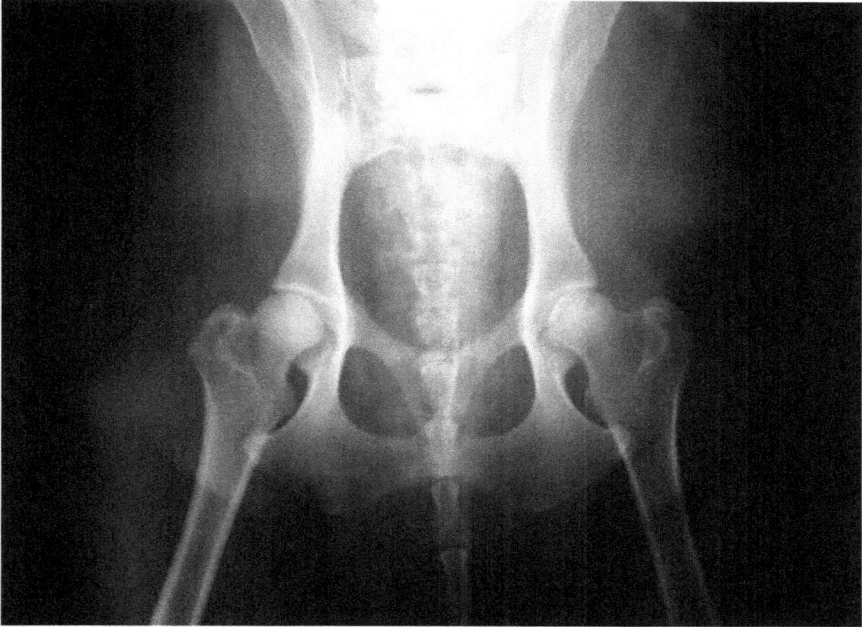

X-ray of normal canine hips.

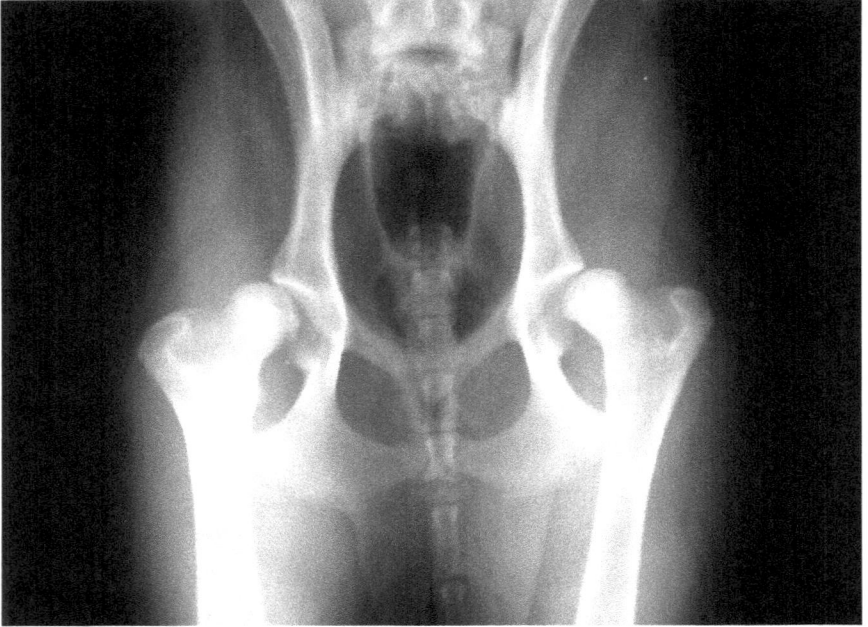

X-ray of canine hips showing dysplasia.

Chapter 3

Western Veterinary Medicine

Every state and country has its own regulations about who can do veterinary acupuncture. Please research the laws before you begin to practice on animals.

I recommend that my dog patients are seen by their vet before I take them on as patients. Since patient history is second-hand (the owner's perspective), western medicine can be very helpful when diagnosing an animal. X-rays, blood tests, etc. may be very useful to help determine what TCM modalities are best to treat the dog. Always find out what medications, supplements and over the counter drugs your dog patient is taking.

It is important to know as much as you can before you prescribe herbs or supplements.

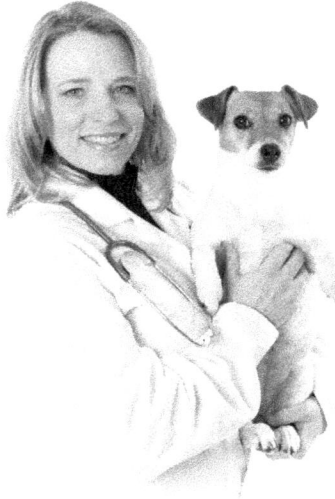

3.1   NSAIDs

Most vets will prescribe non-steroidal drugs (NSAIDS) for pain. The way NSAIDS work is by blocking the body chemicals known as prostaglandins which causes inflammation.

NSAIDS are prescribed to help the following symptoms:

- Joint pain
- Stiffness

- Swelling
- Inflammation

They come in several forms such as pills, drops, caplets, and injections. The most common of the FDA approved NSAIDs are

- Rimadyl (carprofen)
- Metacam (meloxicam)
- Deramax (deracoxib)
- Previcox (firocoxib)
- Novox (generic caprofen)
- Etogesic (etodolac)

Side effects of these drugs include:

- Vomiting
- Change in bowel movements, loose stools, diarrhea, bloody stools, constipation
- Change in behavior
- Depression
- Seizures
- Aggression
- Lack of coordination
- Jaundiced eyes, gums or skin

- Excess thirst
- Change in urination: color, smell, blood in urine, frequency
- Allergic skin reaction, itching, scabs, redness

More serious side effects include:

- Ulcers
- Kidney damage
- Liver problems
- Gastrointestinal bleeding

Owners need to be aware of these potential side effects and contact their veterinarian immediately if the dog is experiencing any of these symptoms. Owners also need to inform their vet of all other medications, herbal supplements, flea and tick control products and over the counter drugs that their dogs are taking.

Never advise a dog owner to reduce or stop any medication the vet has prescribed. This is outside your scope of practice, and is a matter between the patient and the vet.

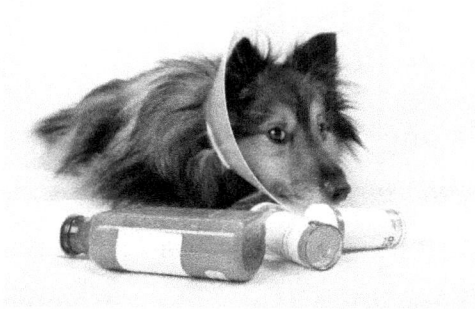

3.2 Opioids

A very popular drug for severe pain is Tramadol (Ultram). Unlike NSAIDs, Tramadol is a synthetic opioid which can be used long term for chronic pain. Like all opiate drugs, withdrawal effects can occur and you owners should be counseled to avoid abruptly stopping the drug if it has been used for very long. In some cases, it may work best when combined with NSAIDs.

It also has side effects , including:

- Constipation (common)
- Whining
- Dog acting drugged or "out of it"
- Excess panting

3.3   Prednisone

Prednisone is one drug that is often used for treating autoimmune diseases, injuries to the spinal cord, inflammation and kidney diseases. It is a synthetic, inactive corticosteroid that is chemically converted by the liver into prednisolone, an active steroid.

Side effects of prednisone include:

- Renal disorders
- Abnormal thirst levels
- Excessive hunger

Side effects that occur after a considerable period of usage may also occur:

- Ulcers in the digestive tract
- Pain and inflammation in pancreas
- Diabetes
- Degeneration of muscles
- Unpredictable change in behaviors

Prolonged use can lead to serious conditions such as Cushing's disease and Addison's disease.

3.4 Adequan

Adequan is an injected substance known as a "poly-sulfated glycosaminoglycan," and is very similar to the oral supplement glucosamine. Adequan has been shown to be absorbed into inflamed joints when injected into a dog's muscles. It soothes and lubricates the joint, naturally reducing inflammation and pain by reducing friction. It actually helps to rebuild cartilage in the damaged joint. Combined with acupuncture this drug is very effective when treating torn ligaments and severe arthritis.

I have found that it is best not to do acupuncture on the same day or even the day after the dog receives an adequan shot as the area is usually tender. Most vets will do the shots 5-6 weeks in a row and then advise one shot a month for maintenance.

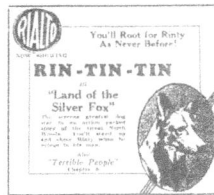

The famous German Shepherd Rin Tin Tin was found as a pup by American serviceman Lee Duncan in France a few months before the end of WWI. He was named after a puppet called Rintintin that French children gave to American soldiers for good fortune. He later went on to star in the TV series Rin Tin Tin.

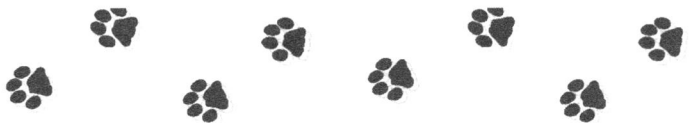

Chapter 4

Acupuncture for Canine Pain

Note: If you are not familiar with point location on animals, there are many similarities between human and animal point locations. As this book is focused on treating canine pain and Bi syndrome, there is only so much basic material I can include. If you are unsure about animal point location, I recommend that you take a basic class before needling an animal for the first time. This is my basic advice for choosing your points.

When choosing which points to needle consider, of course, what points would be the most effective, but balance point selection with the reality that a dog will not allow you to needle many of the points you might use on a human. Sometimes you have to be creative in point selection. For example, some dogs do not like their paws touched let alone needled. Others will not let you needle anywhere near an injury. Some dogs lay on the side that is most painful to protect it. In each of these cases, the selection of alternate points allows the treatment to go forward.

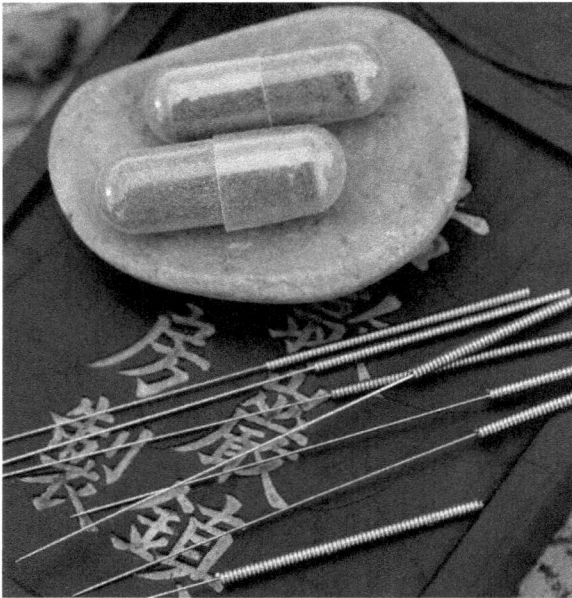

While a human can be warned about a painful point, and may agree to allow its use, a dog has no idea what will happen as a point is needled. Personally, I never needle a point on a dog that I know will cause extreme pain. They never forgive you for it and it makes it more difficult to needle them anywhere else. Dogs usually will allow their back shu points to be needled.

This is my list of points that seem to work the best for arthritic pain. They also generally allow you to treat the dog without getting bit. This is a brief listing: points have several more functions than I show below. For more information about a point refer to your acupuncture texts – point functions are the same between humans and dogs.

Please note that this is a general list, do not use all of these at the same time.

UB 13 Lungs Hollow – Back Shu Point of the Lung. Treats: Pain in the shoulders, neck and upper extremities, lung issues, asthma, allergies; tonifies lung Qi, regulates defensive Wei Qi, stops cough, clears heat.

UB 17 Diaphragm's Hollow – Influential point of Blood. Treats: Vomiting, difficulty swallowing, asthma; tonifies Blood. Use for dogs who are Blood deficient. Calms the mind. Great point for stressed out dogs.

UB 18 Liver's Hollow – Back Shu Point of the Liver. Treats pain in the hypochondriac region, red eyes, epilepsy; Tonifies Liver and Liver Blood. Use for older dogs or those with Liver deficiency. Tonifies the Liver and Gallbladder, moves qi stagnation, cools damp-heat.

UB 23 Kidney's Hollow – Back Shu Point of the Kidney. Treats: Pain and/or weakness in the back, hips, knee and lumbar region, deafness, diarrhea, incontinence, DM; Kidney Yin and or Yang deficiency. Tonifies and regulates Kidney Qi, strengthens the lumbar vertebrae.

UB 28 Bladder's Hollow – Back Shu of the Urinary Bladder. Treats: Pain in the back, hip and lumbar region, UTI, bladder infections, incontinence, hip dysplasia. Regulates the Urinary Bladder, benefits the lumbar vertebrae.

ST 36 Three Mile Run – He-sea Point of the Stomach, Four Sea Point of Nourishment. Treats: Pain in the knee and back, allergies, digestive disorders. Boosts the immune system, tonifies and regulates Blood and Qi. Do not needle if the knee has been operated on recently or if the dog has torn the ACL.

Du 4 Life Gates Fire – Treats: Neck or head pain, bone

pain.

GB 29 Stationary Seam – Treats: Pain of hip and back, paralysis. Use with GB 30 and GB 31 for hip dysplasia.

GB 30 Encircling Leap – Treats: Lumbar pain, hip dysplasia, back and hip pain, muscular atrophy of the lower limbs. Benefits the lower back and legs. Use with GB29 and GB 31 for hip dysplasia.

GB 31 Wind Market – Treats: pain in the hip and lumbar region, hip dysplasia, paralysis of lower limbs. Relaxes muscles, sinews. Strengthens bones. Use with GB29 and GB30 for hip dysplasia.

GB 34 Yang's Tomb Spring – He-Sea point of the Gallbladder, Influential Point of the Tendons. Treats: Muscle pain and injuries, knee problems such as weak knees, pain or swelling in the knees, numbness or pain in lower extremities. Tonifies the Liver and Gallbladder, clears damp-heat, calms rebellious Qi. Do not needle if the knee has been operated on recently or if the dog has torn the ACL.

UB 60 Kunlun Mountains – Jing River Point. Treats: Back pain, UTI, bladder issues. Strengthens the back, relaxes the sinews and muscles, moves Blood and clears heat. Massage UB60 and KI3 together for dogs with back issues.

KI 3 Great Ravine – Yuan Source Point. Treats: Pain in the lower back, knees, asthma, frequent urination. Tonifies Kidney qi, strengthens the knees and lower back.

LI 11 Crooked Pond – He-Sea Point, Tonification Point. Treats: Pain in elbow, front paws, shoulders and upper extremities, allergies and skin problems, febrile diseases.

SI 11 Heavenly Attribution – Treats: Shoulder and upper body pain, asthma, lung problems, coughing.

LI 15 Shoulder Transporting Point – Treats: Movement disorders and pain in the upper extremities, shoulder and neck (use with SJ 14).

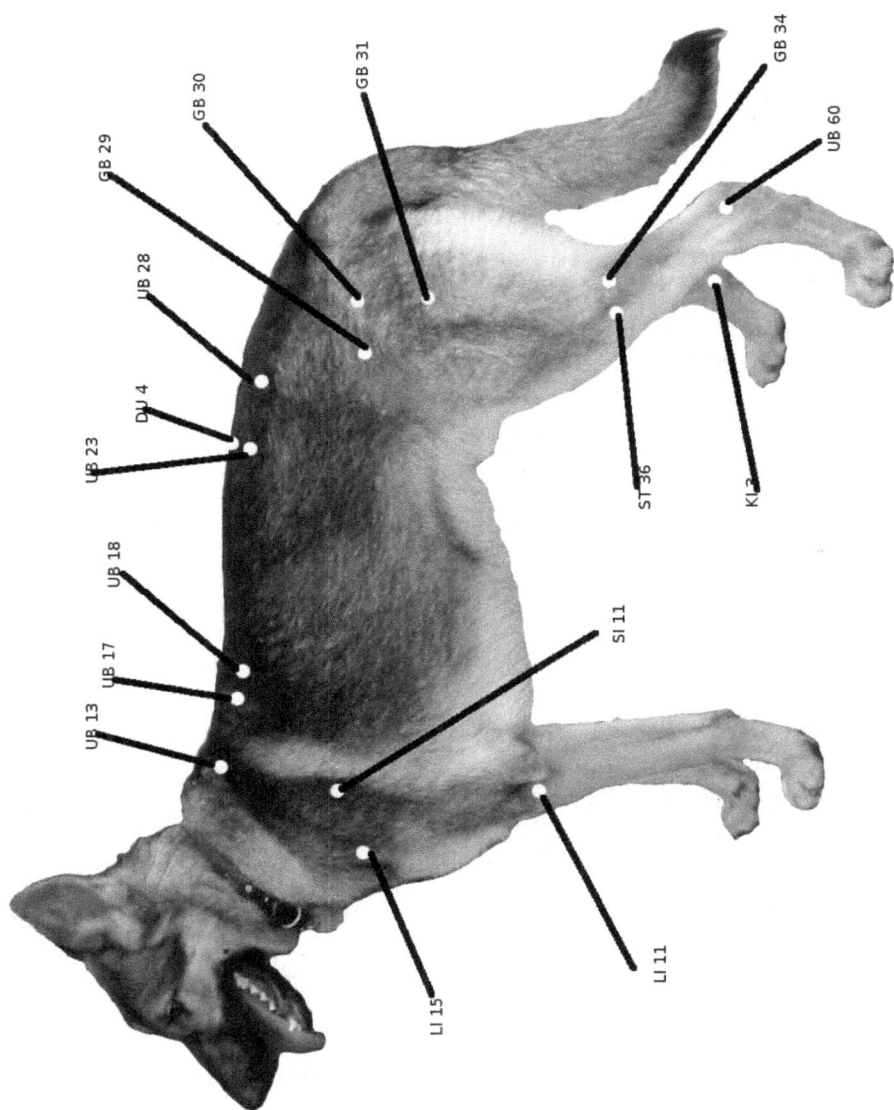

GB 31
GB 30
GB 29
UB 28
DU 4
UB 23
UB 18
UB 17
UB 13
GB 34
UB 60
ST 36
KI 3
SI 11
LI 15
LI 11

4.1   Canine Needle Technique

Dogs are curious and they will often watch the treatment carefully. Before I needle the dog I make sure he or she is calm and comfortable. Needling is usually one of the last things I do in the session. The dog should be in a comfortable place, perhaps his bed or on a carpet in his favorite spot.

Give the dog a nice gentle massage and palpate his spine and any other areas he may be experiencing pain. See if he flinches or yelps at certain points. You may want to do those points last or just laser and massage them if they are too painful.

Some use a thicker gauge needle on a dog but it's not necessary. Why risk increasing the sensation of pain. I prefer to use one inch number 1 Japanese needles (0.16 x 30mm). Do not needle deeply. The dog may roll or move so be sure to stay with the dog at all times.

When opening the needles I allow the dog to sniff them. They all seem curious about them so it is part of my ritual to show them the needles first, tell them that the needles will make them feel good.

A cookie sprayed with Rescue Remedy, a nice pat on

the head with a "good boy" or "good girl" are excellent preludes to needling. As with humans, intention is important when needling your patient. Intention is, after all, Qi. As you needle think of how that point will help the dog or perhaps what the point function is. Or you could visualize the dog feeling happy and painfree. Sometimes this is difficult to do if the owner is a chatter box and keeps talking during the treatment. (Just learn to nod your head and say "mmm hmm" a lot!)

Needle retention depends on what you are treating the dog for and the dog's constitution. Cooperation from the dog is a factor as well. For smaller dogs 10-20 minutes is a blessing. For older dogs, retention from 15-25 minutes is common. Younger dogs and bigger dogs can go up to about 30 minutes, if needed.

When you pull the needles do it gently. After they are pulled praise the dog and thank him or her with a treat. Follow up with a massage or Tui Na with Zheng Gu Shui if needed.

4.2   E-Stim

In acupuncture school, I remember one of my professors was fond of saying that electro-stim is often used to get a bad point prescription to work. I do not use e-stim on dogs, and I have not found it necessary to get excellent results from acupunture.

If choosing to use e-stim on a dog, there are many variables to consider. The main one is this: THEY DON'T LIKE IT!

Another consideration is communication. When you are using e-stim with a human patient you can ask the patient to tell you what they feel and when it is too much. You can't do this with a dog. I once witnessed one of my own dogs scream in pain and try to jump off the table when a vet acupuncturist tried to use e-stim. She was not happy and she never allowed him near her again.

E-stim is indicated for excess conditions. Most of the dogs that I treat are old and deficient, a contraindicated for estim. Rarely do I get a dog who would perhaps benefit from using estim.

E-stim is commonly used by acupuncturist veterinarians. I'm not sure why, except that few have the extensive training in acupuncture that licensed acupuncturist are required to have.

4.3 Laser Acupuncture

Laser acupuncture stimulates the point, increases circulation and reduces inflammation. When working with dogs you cannot always needle some of the points you would on a human. I have found that using a laser to stimulate ashi points and hard to reach points on the dogs is very effective. It is a good way to calm them before needling takes place.

The laser penetrates deep into the skin layers, warming while moving Qi and stimulating the acupuncture point. It provides a mild form of pain relief. I recommend using it up and down meridians for a more effective treatment as well as focusing on each point for at least a few minutes. Most dogs love it and are calmer after the session, making it easier to then needle them.

I use a LED laser which can be found at most acupuncture supply sites. You can opt for a much more expensive clinic laser, but I prefer the handheld laser for use on dogs. You can use it from a bit of a distance if the dog is leery to allow you near him and the dog can also move while you are using it. Ever since I incorporated this laser therapy with acupuncture the treatments have been much more effective.

Make sure to focus the laser on the meridians involved, as well as any acupuncture points you want stimulated. For example: For injuries such as torn ACL, laser around the entire area of the knee as well as the inside of the knee. You can use the laser for the following conditions:

- Arthritis
- Hip Dysplasia
- Muscle Strains
- Elbow and Knee Injuries
- Post-Surgical Recovery
- Wound Healing
- Fractures
- Herniated Disc
- Neck or shoulder pain/injuries

4.4 Infrared Heat Therapy

During cold damp weather using an infrared heat lamp on the dog's back area, hips, knees and elbows is very soothing. Since I make house calls I use a hand held ProM-750 infrared lamp. It is a lightweight, hand held infrared heat lamp. It is perfect for those hard-to-reach areas, on a dog when used with an extension cord.

On cold, damp days I will use the heat lamp over the areas I want to needle just to add some comfort before I actually insert the needle. If I am not doing moxa on the dog I also will hold the heat lamp over the needles to add warmth. The dogs seem to like it so it must feel good!

Warming the joints after massage with a liniment like Zheng Gu Shu helps to ease pain.

4.5 Moxibustion

Moxibustion is the process of burning the herb Artemisia Vulgaris (a type of mugwort) over specific acupuncture points and channels. In theory moxa is great to use on dogs suffering from cold damp bi syndrome. However,

since I make housecalls I have found that many owners are not appreciative of the odor from moxa. Some
dogs do not mind, others run from the smoke. If using
moxa on a dog be very careful to keep the moxa stick
a safe distance from the dog's hair. Often I will give the
owner a lesson on how to use moxa on their dog and
leave them with a moxa stick. Never use direct moxa
or stick-on moxa on a dog.

I was once treating a 17 year old poodle for arthritis
during the dead cold of winter. The dog had stopped
eating, always an ominous sign. However, when I used
moxa on her Stomach 36 her tail would wag. When I
stopped her tail would stop wagging. It provided much
amusement for her owners and after her sessions she
would eat.

4.6   Tui Na

Tui Na is a Chinese system of massage and physical
therapy. Employing the basic principles of acupuncture, combined with modern knowledge of anatomy,
Tui Na is used extensively in China for the treatment
of injuries. Tui Na is also very effective on dogs. After
an acupuncture treatment, while the dog is relaxed, I

like to reward the dog with a round of Tui Na massage, focusing on the areas that are painful as well as the back and hips. I often apply Zheng Gu Shi liniment with Tui Na on dogs.

Take Your Dog to Work Day is the
third Friday of June each year. It was
created to celebrate companions dogs
and to encourage their adoption from
animal shelters, humane societies,
and breed rescue groups.This annual
event asks employers to allow pet lovers
to celebrate their love of dogs and to
promote pet adoption by allowing canines
at their workplace on this one special day.

http://www.takeyourdog.com/About/

Chapter 5

Herbs for Canine Pain

Do your homework before recommending herbal formulas for dogs. Be sure to know all medications the dog is on and be aware of what, if any, drug-herb interactions may take place. The following drugs combined with herbs may cause side effects. Prescribe with caution if the dog is on any of the following types of medications:

- Anticoagulants and anti-platelet drugs
- Diuretics
- Sympathomimetics
- Anti-diabetic drugs
- Cardiac Drugs
- Anti-hypertensive drugs

Note that some herbs that are safe for humans are harmful to dogs. Cats are very sensitive to herbs and this book is geared for treating dogs only. Please do not use these recommended herbal formulas on cats!

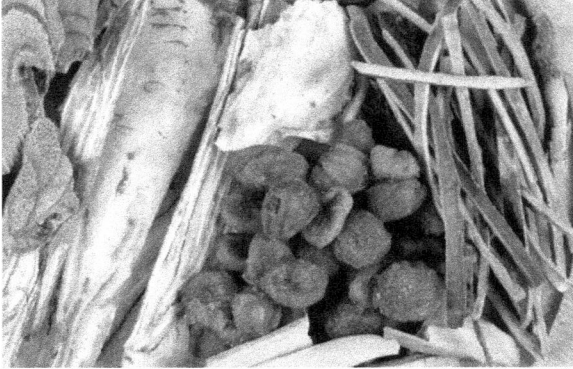

In this book I will only be discussing a few of the many herbal formulas that can be used for dogs suffering from pain symptoms. These are the formulas I use most in my practice and have had the best results from. There are several other excellent formulas to use but in this context there is not enough time to present them all. There are several herbal companies that make these formulas.

For the record, I am not endorsing any company over another. These are examples of products I have used. Each brand of herbal formula has its own interpretation of the original formula so herbs may be added or substituted. When in doubt of what formula to choose for the dog think about what formula you would use if you were treating a human with the same symptoms?

5.1 How to Administer Herbs to Dogs

It can be tricky to get a dog to take medication. Many herbs have a strong smell, especially to dogs. Some are very well behaved and others will be very clever about avoiding anything they don't like. Dogs have been known pretend to take herbs, spitting them out later, and often become masters of extracting an herb tablet from food. Having a few tricks at hand will help you and the owner to more effectively administer herbs.

A few ideas for administering tablets:

- Hide or crush the tablet in the dog's food.
- Wrap the tablet in a piece of meat or cheese.
- Coat the tablet with peanut butter and see if he will take it.
- Roll tablet up in turkey or chicken
- Make a scrambled egg add the tablets right before the egg is completely cooked so the yolk hides the odor and tablet.

More ideas for administering herbal tinctures:

- Add tincture to his portion of wet food.
- Add tincture to rice made with chicken broth or in his daily portion of congee.
- Always praise the dog after the herbs are consumed. Good Boy! Good Girl!

You shouldn't need to say this, but it is important to remind the owners that the herbs need to be taken on a regular basis. Many owners will administer herbs for a few days, then tire of the process and begin skipping doses and days.

Do the Math: Supplement Dosages for Dogs

When you recommend nutritional supplements for a dog, you may only be able to find human versions of the products. That's okay, but be careful about using recommended human dosages. Dosage information for most supplements is based on the needs of an average person of about 125 pounds in weight. To calculate the dog's needs, do the math yourself. For example, to calculate the dosage for a 40 pound dog:

Divide the dog's weight by 125. For example: 40/125 = .32

Multiply the recommended dosage by this number: For example: 3 tablets, twice per day. 3 X .32 = .96.

So, rounding the final number a bit, the dosage of this supplement for a 40 pound dog would be 1 tablet, twice per day.

5.2   Treating Cold Damp

My favorite formula for treating dogs with symptoms made worse by cold damp weather is: Du Huo Jisheng Wan (Angelica pubescens and Sangjisheng decoction aka Supple Spine in the Kan Essentials for Animals).

This formula I use a lot in the winter and early spring here in New England. When doing an intake always try to determine if the dog's symptoms are made worse by weather conditions. Have the owner write any symptoms down on a calendar along with the weather that day. Usually there is a connection. I have found on very cold damp days most of my older dog patient's symptoms are worse.

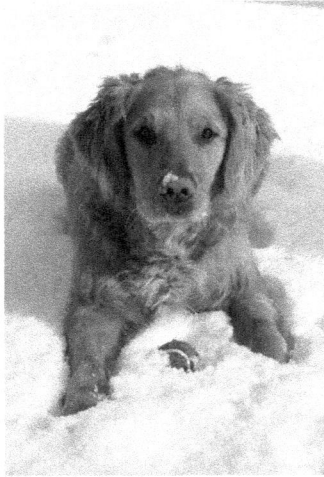

For lower back, hip or knee pain made worse by cold damp weather, I often use this formula. Usually the diagnosis includes symptoms of kidney qi, yin and or yang deficiency. This is a great formula for older dogs suffering from arthritis. Symptoms may include:

- Pain in the lower back, hip region
- Pain in knees and/or elbows
- Difficulty getting up
- Stiffness in legs
- Aversion to cold damp or symptoms worse on cold damp days

Older dogs usually have a combination of kidney qi, yin and yang deficiency. Symptoms may include:

- Deafness
- Confusion
- Fatigue
- Tired eyes
- Weak hind quarters
- Lameness after exercise
- Muscle spasms especially in the back
- White muzzle
- Profuse urination
- Constipation or loose stools
- Slow, labored walking
- They look old!

When treating a dog with these symptoms I not only do acupuncture but I also use an infrared hand held lamp applied to their back, knees, elbows and hips. Most dogs like this. I also use a laser on points they usually will not let me needle.

Along with the herbal formula for cold damp please remind the owner to keep the dog warm in colder weather. Make sure the dog's bed is not in a drafty area. If the dog likes to be covered leave a blanket near his bed or cover him. Several companies now make dog coats and sweaters that will keep the dog warmer. Dogs with shorter fur, (like black labs) may be more affected by cold damp weather.

Du Huo Ji Sheng Wan Ingredients

(Angelica Pubescens and Sangjisheng Decoction)

Table 5.1: Du Huo Ji Sheng Wan Ingredients

Radix Angelicae Pubescentis
Herba cum Radice Asari
Radix Ledebouriellae Divaricatae
Radix Gentianae Qinjiao
Ramulus Sangjisheng
Cortex Eucommiae Ulmoidis
Radix Achyranthus Bidentatae
Cortex Cinnamoni Cassiae
Radix Angelicae Sinensis
Radix Ligustici Chuanxiong
Radix Rehmanniae Glutinosae
Radix Paeoniae Lactiflorae
Radix Ginseng
Sclerotium Poriae Cocos
Honey-fried Radix Glycyrrhizae Uralenisis

Actions: expels wind-dampness, disperses painful obstruction and tonifies deficiency.

Once again remind the owners that herbs must be administered on a regular basis and they may not see any positive results for a week or so. Do NOT not use this formula when it is hot and humid out.

Case History

An example of a dog who would need this formula is Chula, a 11 year old shepherd lab mix who lives in Boston. She has stiffness in the back and knees, worsened by cold, rain and winter. Sometimes she needs help getting up after a nap. She is losing her hearing. Her muzzle is turning white. She is a very good natured dog and loves her stuffed squirrel and cookies.

Along with the herbal formula her owner changed her diet to home-cooked congee with brown rice during the cold months, and changed to a brand of dry dog food that is free of wheat, corn and soy. In the summer she is fed a healthy brand of wet dog food along with dry food. Her owner massages Zheng Gu Shui liniment into her back, knees and hips once a day after her nightly walk. He added carpet runners on the hardwood floor to make it easier for her to walk and to keep the floor warmer in the winter. Chula received acupuncture once a week for six weeks, regaining much of her energy and movement. Treatments continued every 4-6 weeks thereafter.

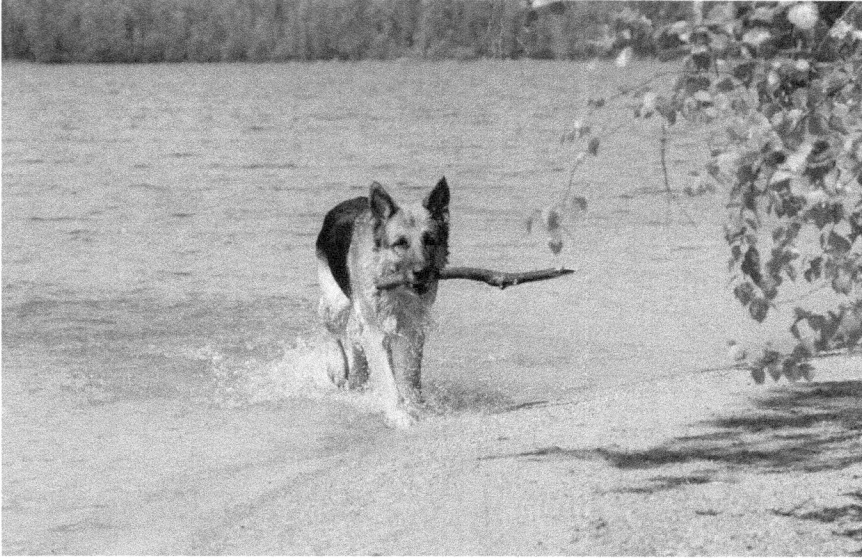

5.3 Treating Damp Heat

Xian Fang Huo Ming Yin (sublime formula for sustaining life) is a formula used for damp heat accumulation. Originally this formula was used for fire toxin pathogens, and has been used as an antimicrobial for infections.

This is the formula for the hot stinky overweight dog that limps!

Symptoms of Damp Heat

- Heat intolerance
- Overweight
- Pain worse during damp humid wet weather
- Stinky pus or oozing
- Dog's symptoms get worse with rest or over exertion
- The dog may also have:
- Infected wounds
- Abscesses
- Hot red lesions
- Inflamed tumors
- Lameness

This is a dog that needs to be kept cool. In the summer help the dog stay cool by providing access to a cool room with plenty of water. A proper diet is very important to help overweight dogs. As with humans, arthritis and other joint pain is worsened by having to carry extra weight.

Xian Fang Huo Ming Yin Ingredients

(Sublime Formula for Sustaining Life)

Actions: Clears heat and relieves fire toxin, reduces

Table 5.2: Xian Fang Huo Ming Yin Ingredients

Flos Lonicerae Japonicae
Radix Glycyrrhizae Uralensis
Blubus Fritilariae Thubergii
Radix Trichosanthis Kirilowii
Radix Angelicae Sinensis
Radix Paeoniae Rubrae
Gummi Olibanum
Myrrha
Radix Ledebourieellae Divaricatae
Radix Angelicae Dahuricae
Squama Manitis Pentadactylae
Spina Gleditsiae
Pericarpium Citri Reticulatae

swelling and promotes the discharge of pus, invigorates blood and alleviates pain.

Case History

An example of a dog who would use this formula is JJ, an overweight black lab that will consume any food left laying around the house. He has been known to open the refrigerator while his owners are gone and eat mass quantities of whatever he can reach. His vet has recommended that he lose 15 pounds.

JJ has been diagnosed with arthritis. He limps on occasion. He has a yellow discharge in his eyes in the morning and a few hot spots on his elbows. He stinks too! He has gas and loose stools. His owners use a cheap dog food found in the grocery store along with table scraps and an occasional donut. JJ becomes worse during a hot muggy summer day and hides under the porch to stay cool.

Besides taking this formula, the first thing that needed to be addressed was JJ's weight and diet. The owner reluctantly switched to a higher quality dog food and attempted to barricade the refrigerator and trash compactor that JJ raided while she was away. He was allowed to stay in the room with AC in the summer. JJ improved steadily with these changes and regular administration of the herbal formula. Eventually he did lose some weight. He received acupuncture 5 weeks in a row with a once a month session for a tune up.

5.4 Kidney Yin and Liver Xue Deficiency

Liu Wei Di Huang Wan (six ingredient pill with rehmannia) is a formula that is great for older dogs who show signs of kidney and liver yin deficiency. Many of these dogs do not do well in hot weather. They have red dry tongues with little or no coat. They may pant and pace at night or are restless. They may like to lay on a cold floor or a cool spot. Sometimes you can actually feel the heat coming off the dog's spine when you palpate. This is for a hot (though deficient) dog! This formula tonifies yin and nourishes the kidneys. Symptoms include:

- Weak and or pain of lower back
- Diminished hearing
- Panting
- Incontinence at night
- Hot to the touch
- Prefers cool spots
- Symptoms worse in hot weather
- Grey muzzle

This dog should also be kept in a cool room, have plenty of water and cooling foods. In diet, avoid beef, as it is a warming meat that contributes to these symptoms.

Liu Wei Di Huang Wan Ingedients

(Six Ingredient Pill with Rehmannia)

Table 5.3: Liu Wei Di Huang Wan Ingredients

Radix Rehmanniae Glutinosae Conquitae
Fructus Corni Officinalis
Radix Dioscoreae Opposiatae
Sclerotium Poriae Cocos
Cortex Noutan Radicis
Rhizoma Alismatis Orientalis

Actions: Enriches the yin and nourishes the kidneys.

Case History

Lady is a 14 year-old big, fluffy, mixed breed dog. She suffers from back and hip pain, lost most of her hearing, has cataracts, pants heavily and is up most of the night driving her owner crazy by pacing in the bedroom. She is also incontinent. She lays on the cold floor even in winter. Her muzzle is partially white and grey and she walks like an old lady. She is worse in hot weather.

Lady responded positively to acupuncture after the first session. Her eyes became brighter and her hair even perked up. Her owner took her off store-bought dog food and began to cook for her. She also added Smart Water (water with electrolytes) to her bowl along with Rescue Remedy, and started her on the herbal formula right away. The only complaint about the formula was that it caused gas. This was remedied by reducing the dose and adding probiotics into her food.

Lady's incontinence did not go away completely but it was reduced to only a few nights a week with the occasional accident. She received acupuncture for 6 consecutive weeks, then received further treatment on an as-needed basis until she passed away at the age of 16.5 years.

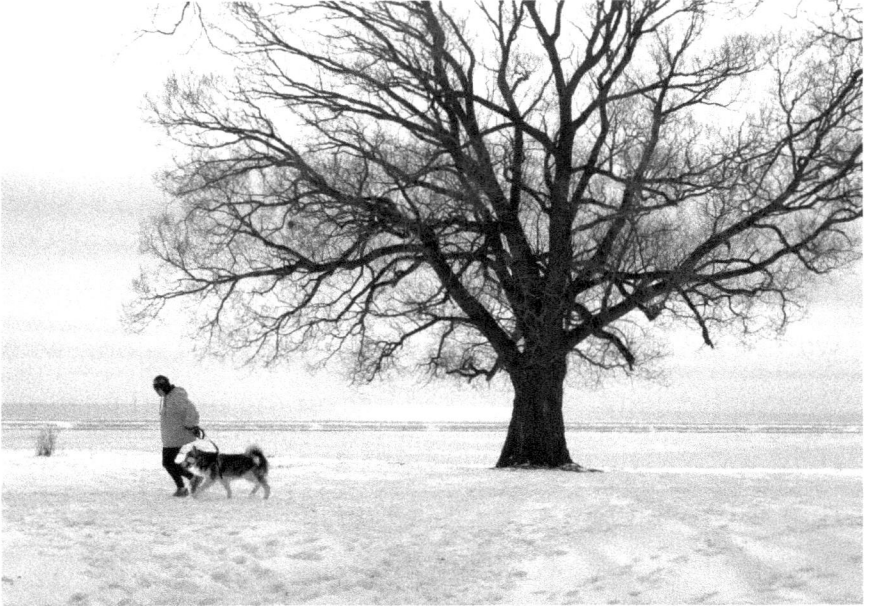

5.5   Treating Kidney Yang Xu

You Gui Wan (Restore the Right Kidney Pill) is a great formula for older dogs who's symptoms worsen in winter. This is an effective formula for dogs with Kidney Yang Xu , hip dysplasia, renal failure, arthritis made worse with cold, degenerative myelopathy and similar conditions. Symptoms include:

- Aversion to cold
- Incontinence both bowel and urinary
- Loose stools

- Sore lower back, knees hips
- Weakness in hips back and knees
- Cold extremities
- Edema of lower extremities
- Acting confused or disoriented

This dog would benefit from infrared heat therapy, moxa, warming foods, and a nice cozy warm bed away from drafts.

You Gui Wan Ingredients

(Restore the Right Kidney Pill)

Table 5.4: You Gui Wan Ingredients

Radix Laterais Aconiti Carmichaeli Praeparata
Cortex Cinnamomi Cassiae
Colla Cornu Cervi
Radix Rehmaanniae Glutinosae Conquitae
Fructus Corni Officinalis
Radix Dioscoreae Oppositae
Fructus Lycii
Semen Cuscutae Chinensis
Cortex Eucommiae Ulmoidis
Radix Angelicae Sinensis

Actions: Warms and tonifies the Kidney Yang, replenishes the Essence and tonifies the Blood.

Note: You can now find dog bones made from the antlers of Cornu Cervi in some of the better pet shops. These are excellent Kidney Yang treats for dogs!

Case History

Bear is a 11 year old purebred German Shepherd, diagnosed with hip dysplasia and arthritis, a common ailment for German Shepherd dogs. His muzzle is turning white and at times he seems disoriented. He is losing his hearing and has cloudy eyes. He took a turn for the worse in the winter. When in pain he will lay in the same spot until someone helps him up. Recently he has become incontinent and is unaware of bowel movements.

Bear received 6 consecutive treatments with little improvement. It was not until the 7th that we turned the corner. Quite surprisingly, he was able to get up and walk normally. Even his face seemed to brighten. Bear was one of my best patients. He allowed me to needle what ever points I wanted and he fell asleep during his sessions. In his point formula, I used a combination of

Du 20 with the tip of the tail point for him. It seemed to be that combo that worked best.

By then too his owner had changed his food, began massaging him with Zheng Gu Shui liniment daily, and moved his bed to a warmer part of the house. Bear continued to make positive progress and lived a very happy life until he was 13.5 years old. The formula You Gui Wan helped keep the incontinence at bay. Occasionally there were accidents in the house, however it was not until his last month of life that the accidents became daily and the herbs no longer seemed to help.

5.6 Chinese Herbal Liniments

After I have pulled my acupuncture needles, I end the dog's treatment with Tui Na to the painful areas, often using the liniment Zheng Gu Shui. Since it contains no oils, like the liniment Po Sum On, it is safe for the dog, and it feels good. Sometime dogs do not like the smell or will sneeze. I recommend the use of a spray bottle. Spray Zheng Gu Shui lightly on the area before administering massage. Do not spray too much: you want enough to soak through the fur but not too much, as it may cause a rash. Areas I often use the Zheng Gu

Shui and massage technique include the knees, back, hips, elbows, and neck. If the dog is afraid of spray bottles, pour a small amount of the Zheng Gu Shui on a clean wash cloth and gently rub it on the affected area.

Be sure not to spray this liniment near any orifices, cuts, open wounds or hot spots. Wash your hands after the massage. If you have any paper cuts or open wounds wear gloves. Zheng Gu Shui is also available in a roll-on bottle. Do not use it. The liquid is poorly regulated, and too much liquid often comes out of it, risking skin irritation.

Another safe liniment to use is Dit Dat Jow. It does not penetrate as well as Zheng Gu Shui, but it does not cause irritation and there is less concern about using too much. Administer it using the same method as Zheng Gu Shui.

Whichever liniment you choose, the owner should watch you and learn to administer it to the dog at least once a day. The best time is after the dog has been outside, but not right before a walk.

The Dog is one of the 12 animals which appear in the Chinese zodiac and calendar.

Dates of the Chinese Year of the Dog:

* 1898 - 2 February 1899: Earth Dog
* 10 February 1910 - 21 January 1911: Metal Dog
* 28 January 1922 - 14 February 1923: Water Dog
* 14 February 1934 - 25 January 1935: Wood Dog
* 2 February 1946 - 21 January 1947: Fire Dog
* 17 February 1958 - 8 February 1959: Earth Dog
* 6 February 1970 - 26 January 1971: Metal Dog
* 25 January 1982 - 12 February 1983: Water Dog
* 10 February 1994 - 30 January 1995: Wood Dog
* 29 January 2006 - 17 February 2007: Fire Dog
* 16 February 2018 - 4 February 2019: Earth Dog

Chapter 6

Supplements and Lifestyle

Herbal formulas are not the only remedies to help ease pain and stress in dogs. Sometimes owners are not willing to give their dogs herbs or the dog may be on so much medication that giving him an herbal supplement is not an option.

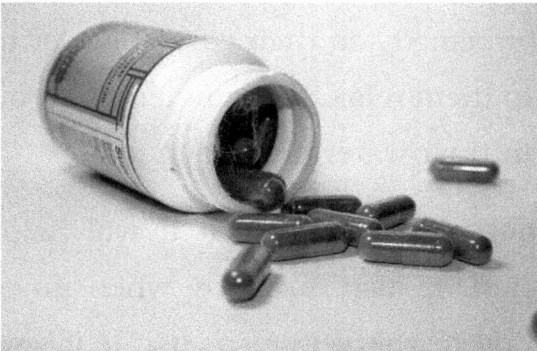

Here are some of the supplements I recommend. All can be found on line or in most stores like Whole Foods or The Vitamin Shoppe.

6.1   Bach Flower Rescue Remedy®

This is one of my favorite remedies to use for animals. Though this remedy does not treat physical pain, I recommend Rescue Remedy to all my patients so their dogs can be more relaxed. Stress relief aids in the healing process. I also recommend this remedy to dog owners who are stressed or worried about their animal.

Bach Flower Rescue Remedy is a mixture of five of the Bach Original Flower Essences. It has an immediate calming effect on pets, especially in stressful situations. To administer, I usually spray a dog cookie and give it to the dog before a treatment. You can also massage the remedy on their ears, paws or top of their head to help them relax. I recommend that owners add 2-3 drops in their water bowl each day.

This will not reduce pain, but it will help with the stress of pain. It also is handy when an owner has to take a dog to the vet. Also, use it if your dog patient has fear of loud noises or other similar situations (fireworks, etc.).

The original Bach Rescue Remedy Ingredients

- Impatiens: Lowers stress
- Star of Bethlehem: For trauma and shock
- Cherry Plum: For those who fear losing control
- Rock Rose: For situations in which one experiences panic or terror.
- Clematis: For those who find their lives unhappy and withdraw into themselves

Bach Flower also makes single flower remedies for specific emotions and behaviors. You can visit their website for more information on those: www.bachflower.com.

6.2   Omega 3 Essential Fatty Acids

An Omega 3 essential fatty acid supplement from cold water oily fish such as salmon, herring, mackerel, anchovies and sardines is best. Flax seed oil contains Omega 3 acids.

Omega 3 fatty acid works as an anti-inflammatory. It helps to lubricate the joints and reduce inflammation.

Omega 3 oils will also improve the health and appearance of your dog's coat, and have been shown to help reduce excess weight in people and dogs.

Most dogs like the taste of fish or flax oil. If you cannot find a brand for pets you can use fish oil in capsules by cutting it open and drizzling it in their food. Begin with low doses, as these supplements can cause gas or loose stools when overused.

6.3   Wobenzym®

Wobenzym® is a natural anti-inflammatory and immune support formula It is a non-prescription formula for acute injuries, chronic joint conditions, infections, and post-operative recovery.

This supplement formula contains a blend of pancreatin, trypsin, chymotrypsin, bromelain, papain, and rutin. These substances are often used as digestive aids, but Wobenzym is taken between meals on an empty stomach and its enteric coating protects these ingredients until they are released in the small intestine, where they do the most good. From the small intestine, they move throughout the body, reducing inflammation wherever it occurs by breaking harmful proteins into smaller chains of amino acids. This type of treatment is known as systemic oral enzyme therapy.

There is a product you may find called Fido-Wobenzym. This is a canine-specific formulation, but it has a potentially harmful red dye in it and is banned in Germany. I prefer to use the human grade Wobenzym to stay on the safe side.

Please note as a precaution that Wobenzym's combination of enzymes can thin the blood. Wobenzym is not recommended for dogs with bleeding or clotting disorders or for any animal on medication that causes blood thinning. Start off with smaller dosage to avoid loose stools or diarrhea in sensitive dogs.

6.4 Glucosamine, Chondroitin and MSM

Glucosamine with MSM (methylsulfonylmethane) helps protect and lubricate joints. Research has shown that MSM has an strong anti-inflammatory effect. Glucosamine has been studied for over 20 years in humans, and has been shown effective to relieve arthritic joint pain.

Please note that it may take four to six weeks before your dog feels the results from these supplements. There are several wonderful brands made specifically for dogs.

6.5   Homeopathic Remedies

Even though homeopathic remedies are not part of Traditional Chinese Medicine, there are a few I recommend for treating pain and stress. The products listed below are safe for humans, dogs and cats and can be taken with medication. You can find these at most health food stores, vitamin shops and online.

Calms Forte® by Hylands

Calms Forte® is a homeopathic remedy for humans used to sooth and ease nervous tension and irritation. It is used to help with sleep disorders, stress and strain. It does not cause drowsiness or strange behavior.

I found this inexpensive remedy very helpful when my 19 year old cat was having difficulty sleeping and resting comfortably in the last few months of her life. The tablets are small and can be dissolved into water or food. I also use this remedy when my dog is having a panic attack at night during a thunderstorm (I combine this with Rescue Remedy and the Thundershirt to keep her calm and it works!). Depending on the animal's weight I vary the amount to give. My fifteen pound cat was given one per night while my 65 pound dog is given two.

Arnica Montana 30X

This homeopathic remedy should be in everyone's medicine cabinet. It relieves the symptoms of muscle pain, soreness, bruising and swelling due to injuries and overexertion. It is a safe and natural pain reliever that can be given to dogs for pain. It will not interfere with medication and can be used everyday. I like the Hylands 30x since the tablets can be dissolved into water or the pet's food.

6.6 Lifestyle Changes for Dog Owners

As I try to explain to my clients, not only does their dog benefit from a combination of acupuncture, herbs, supplements and a change of diet, sometimes a simple lifestyle change can make a major difference in the dog's healing process. Here are some of the recommendations I give:

When Fleas Invade

One of the hazards of making house-calls is that you may bring home fleas. Not all pet owners are conscientious about keeping their homes flea free. Here is an inexpensive and easy remedy to recommend to your clients.

To rid your home of fleas, get a box of 20 Mule Team Borax (available in your grocery store laundry aisle), and spread it lightly over your carpet. Use a broom to sweep it deeply into the carpet. Wait a couple of hours then vacuum. The residual Borax that remains in the carpet will kill the fleas and their larvae simply by drying them out. Make sure your pets do not walk on the floor while the Borax is there. It can be absorbed into their feet. When washing dog beds, towels and sheets sprinkle Borax on them before washing as a precaution to kill any eggs that might be hiding in the fibers.

Aromatherapy for Pests

April showers bring May flowers with fleas, ticks and other bugs that attack our pets.

Ticks carry the dreaded Lyme disease as well as yellow-spotted fever disease and other nasty diseases, some of them very dangerous for dogs. Fleas are annoying to both humans and animals and can cause serious disease.

Many people have asked me about recommendations for natural pest repellents for their dogs. There are a few essential oils that can help combat ticks and fleas, however there is no guarantee that these aromatherapy mixtures will completely protect your dog. Always err on the side of caution when bringing your dog into an area that is known to have ticks. Use whatever products, natural or otherwise, that are needed to protect your pet.

Here are a few essential oils to make your own *Pest Away Repellent*:

Please note that certain aromatherapy oils are toxic for cats. The following essential oils are for human or dog use only.

- Geranium oil is said to be one of the best oils to repel ticks and fleas. It can also be used as a hair and skin conditioner.
- Lavender oil is soothing, calming and repels most bugs, ticks and even scorpions.

- Lemongrass repels ticks, fleas and mosquitoes.
- Sage and thyme are also used with other oils to repel ticks.

To make your own essential oil repellent, take about 4 drops of one or more of the above oils mixed into 8 ounces of pure water in a dark glass spray bottle. You can use this mixture on your dog, the dog's bedding and even yourself! Please be careful not to spray near eyes or any orifices (yours or the dog's).

Music Sooths the Savage Beast

Many of my clients are stunned when I insist that all TV, radio and music must be turned off in the house during their dog's acupuncture session. Music has a very powerful effect on all of us. Calming and classical music has been proven to relax people as well as animals. Loud or angry music agitates both people and dogs. Have you ever notice that you become agitated while shopping in a store playing annoyingly loud music? Perhaps you would have stayed and shopped longer if the music was happy, peaceful or classical? Have you ever tried to eat in a restaurant that had really bad booming music?

A dog's sense of hearing is their second most developed organ. They can hear frequencies into the ultrasound and infrasound range. Dogs can hear things humans can't even fathom! So can you even imagine what booming loud music does to them – especially music with lots of heavy base like rap or heavy metal. It is upsetting, disturbing and can make them very cranky! (It does the same to people too.)

If I am treating a very sensitive dog on a house call I bring my own music. When working at the vet's office I also bring a small boom box to play in my room. (I also ask that all other music that is usually piped into the room be turned off.)

You can play classical or relaxing music during your sessions. One of my favorite CDs to play is from the CD *Through a Dog's Ear*. The music has been clinically tested on dogs and cats, and shown to create a relaxation response. I play it in my house for my own animals whenever I am away. My husband, also an acupuncturist plays this CD for his human patients. Everyone seems to chill out when listening to concert musician Lisa Spector play these classical melodies. I recommend this music to my clients to play when their pets are stressed. Put on repeat mode when away for the day or play in the car for long trips. It's a nice alternative to playing the TV or radio.

Through a Dog's Ear

www.ThroughADogsEar.com

800-788-0949

6.7   The Thundershirt®

When I first learned about the Thundershirt®, I have to admit I thought it was a hoax. After we adopted our dog Quan Yin, a rescue abandoned in the 2010 floods of Tennessee we had no idea what to expect. A sweet natured girl who loves to be loved, however just the prediction of a thunderstorm several miles away had her shaking and hiding. No amount of Rescue Remedy, Valerian or Bach Flowers could calm her completely. That is when we surrendered and tried a Thundershirt. Viola! The shirt combined with Rescue Remedy has made Quan Yin a much calmer dog. And made me a believer!

If you are not familiar with this new product let me try to explain what it is. The Thundershirt is literally a shirt that you wrap around your dog or cat. It comes in sizes and has easy Velcro fasteners so it can be fitted to your pet.

Wrapping your dog or cat in this swaddling material helps calm it during thunder storms, fireworks and stressful situations. It works by applying constant, gentle pressure which calms your dog. Sounds so simple. Yes — it is. I now highly recommend this product to patients suffering from extreme fear and stress.

You can learn more about the Thundershirt at:

www.thundershirt.com or call 866-892-2078.

If you would like to carry this product in your clinic the folks at Thundershirt can help you do that too.

Add Carpets and Runners on Hard Wood Floors

This is one of my pet peeves!

So many times I have treated dogs who were unable to get up from or stand on bare floors because there was no rug under them to add traction. Hip and leg problems, and old age, make bare floors very difficult for a dog. Unfortunately there are dog owners who are not happy about having "unsightly" rugs in their designer rooms, even if it makes a major difference in their dog's life.

I once treated an AKC Blue Ribbon famous Sheepdog whose owner was a wealthy antique dealer in New England. Her house was decorated as if it were in a Home & Garden magazine. Shiny hardwood floors, pricey art and not a comfortable spot in the entire house for the dog (or human). The vet had referred this patient to me as he had given up any hope to help this poor aging dog, suffering from severe arthritis and weak knees. For the sake of this story let's just call the dog Fluffy. Fluffy's owner thought that one acupuncture session would instantly heal her dog. When I recommended adding carpets and runners on the floor where Fluffy frequently walked, the owner's response was: "That is not an option." A few more visits to the home, Fluffy was really not responding to the treatments. The owner would not follow any of the recommendations given. She refused to change the food, to administer herbal supplements and the smell of the Zheng Gui Shu liniment "stunk"!

As I watched Fluffy struggle to get up from the slippery floor I once again brought up the idea of adding runners again to help Fluffy. The answer was a resounding "No!" As a result, I told the owner she was wasting my time and her money and contacted the veterinarian. He also tried to convince the owner that a few runners would make a difference for Fluffy only to receive a negative response. Another owner chose to "put his dog down" rather than put a few carpet runners on the floor. I guess this experience is one that will always stay in my mind with a huge question mark hovering over it. Why was it so hard to just lay out a rug for the poor dog? Of course, this is one of those people that will say they tried acupuncture but it did not work! Sadly, there are many stories like these. Too many.

Add Runners On Wooden Stairs

Another common sense solution for a dog who is having difficulty going up or down the stairs. Once a dog has a bad experience going down a slippery flight of stairs he may never want to try it again. Adding a carpet runner or pads can help.

Weather and Temperature

Keep the dog warm in winter. Make sure his bed is not near a drafty area. Provide a warm bed, blankets and pillows. If it is a dog who is suffering from pain made worse from Cold Damp you may want to have a space heater near by or leave the heat on. Keep food and water near by.

In the summer make sure the dog is kept cool and has plenty of water. If you are leaving the dog outside provide a weatherproof dog house he can stay in. Make sure it is in the shade. Inside the house leave a fan or air conditioner on. These seem like common sense ideas, but are often forgotten in the a dog owner's busy life.

Seven Tips to Cool Off A Hot Dog

- *PLEASE! Never, ever leave your pets in a parked car in the summer, even if you crack the windows or park in the shade. A car temperature can rise to 150F or more in just a few minutes. This is the number one cause of canine heat stroke.*

- *Always have plenty of fresh water handy for your pets. Carry a bottle of water and a bowl for your dog when walking him or her on a hot day. Add SmartWater to your dog's bowl which has electrolytes and can help prevent dehydration.*

- *Be on the look-out for signs of heatstroke. Symptoms include rapid breathing, a dazed look, very hot skin and twitching muscles. Wrap your pet in a cool, but NOT cold, wet towel. Get them to the vet as soon as possible as heatstroke can be fatal.*

- *Be careful not to exercise dogs during the hottest part of the day. Also don't worry if they are eating less on hot days as it is a normal canine reaction to heat.*

- *Put a kiddie pool for dogs to cool off and play in on those hot summer days. They are inexpensive and can be found at most stores like Target.*

- *Try to keep your pets indoors during the hottest part of the day, in a room with air conditioning or circulating fans if possible.*

- *Short haired dogs or those who have just been shaved are prone to sunburn just like us. Especially early in the summer, try to limit your dog's exposure to the sun.*

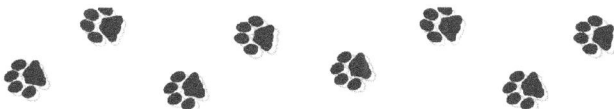

Chapter 7

Nutrition

Nutrition is as important to dogs as it is for humans. "You are what you eat" applies to our four pawed friends as well. Good Nutrition plays a major part in treating a dog suffering from pain related syndromes. If a dog is overweight and is suffering from arthritis, hip or elbow dysplasia, or a torn ACL, it is important for the dog to lose weight to ease the pain and burden of the weight on his limbs.

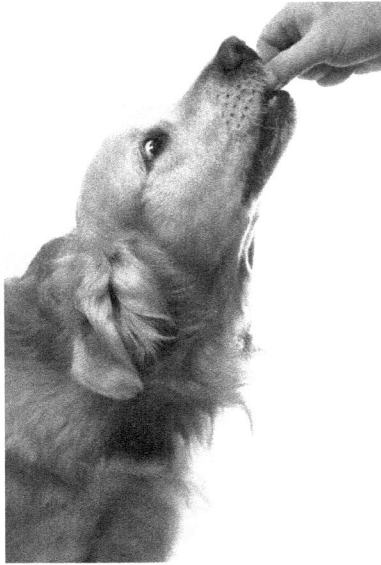

Here is the advice I give to all clients:

First, it's important to know what NOT to feed your dog. Research has shown that wheat aggravates the symptoms of arthritis and most pain. Make sure you feed your dog food that does not contain fillers, by products, wheat, soy or corn. Unfortunately wheat gluten is used in several name brand pet foods. Wheat also is a major factor in weight. Once you eliminate the wheat in a dog's diet you may notice that he is in less pain, may lose weight and if he has allergies they may be eliminated.

Read the label and avoid using brands that contain the following:

- Animal meat meal and animal by-products – this is what is left of the slaughtered animal after the meat is removed. It can include things like beaks, feet, blood, intestines, bones, and tissue .

- Beef and bone meal – another by product of beef which can include hair, hooves, horn, manure, entrails and blood.

- Corn bran – which is the outer layer of the corn kernel. It has no nutritional value.

- Corn Gluten – is the residue from corn which can be used as a protein but can cause allergies in many dogs just like wheat gluten.

Most of the common brands in the grocery store are not good. They have fillers, preservatives, and are hard to digest. After the pet food recall of 2007 more people are willing to pay a bit extra for pet food that is safe.

I recommend buying brands that use free-range meats or fish. Meat that is not free range may contain antibiotics and hormones which are harmful to both humans and animals. If you are going to feed the dog wet food I would recommend a combination of both wet and dry.

Just like people, dogs should be fed at the same time everyday, if possible. When switching to a new brand or cooked food there should be a transition process. Often, switching foods confuses the dog (though some dogs will eat anything!) and a change in food may cause either diarrhea, loose stools or even constipation.

I recommend the process below to introduce new food into the diet:

During the first week of switching use about 75% of the old food and 25% of the new.

Second week: Use 50% of the old food and 50% of the new.

Third week: 25% of the old and 75% of the new.

Fourth week 100% all new food.

7.1   Bloat

Larger dogs are prone to bloat (canine gastric delation volvulus - CGDV). Bloat is a very dangerous, life-threatening condition.

It occurs when the dog is swallowing air while gulping down a large meal. Exercising too soon after a meal is a contributing factor. It can also occur if the dog drinks too much water too quickly.

The stomach then swells with fluid and gas, then begins to twist. This traps the gas inside causing the blood supply to the digestive organs to shut off. The dog will act as if in pain, and is stomach will be taut and swollen. The dog must be immediately rushed to a veterinarian or he or she can go into shock and die.

When feeding dogs, owners of large breeds should be aware of the risks of bloat, and control the amount and frequency of feeding to avoid it.

7.2 Cooking for Your Dog

Whenever possible I recommend cooking for a dog who is old and in pain. A cooked meal is tonifying, healthier and the dog feels more satisfied after eating. Many dogs will stop begging while their owners are eating if they have been fed a home-cooked meal. It is less expensive in the long run to cook for your dog. You can use a crock pot or a rice cooker and make enough food for a few days.

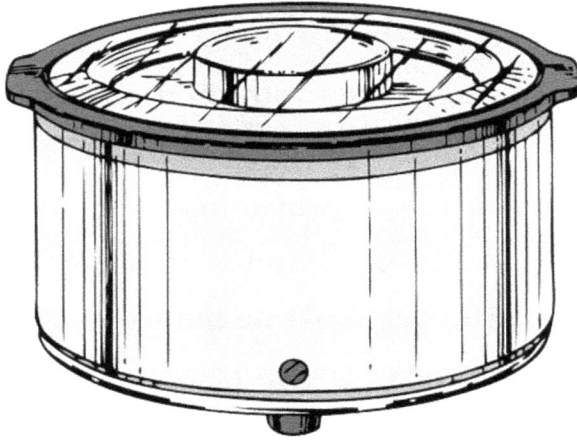

There are several opinions on cooking for your dog versus feeding your dog a raw diet sometimes known as the BARF (Biologically appropriate raw food diet). Raw diets are based on the concept that naturally, in the wild, canines eat raw meat. However, our dogs are far removed from their wild beginnings. Also, the raw meat eaten by dogs in the wild is quite different than the meat we get from the over-processed, drug enhanced, antibiotic laden meat you'll find at your local grocery.

From a TCM point of view a raw diet will damage the spleen. If an owner chooses a raw diet they must make sure the dog is getting proper amounts of vegetables or greens along with the meat. In the wild dogs would eat grass or herbs to aid in digestion after consuming their prey. Dogs on the BARF diet should be fed fresh organic meats only to avoid the risk of Salmonella or other diseases contracted by eating raw food.

Congee Recipe for your Dog

We all know there is nothing like a home cooked meal. Here is a recipe for those dogs who suffer from arthritis, hip dysplasia and other ailments, especially those made worse by damp weather.

This is the recipe I used for my dog Merlin, a German Shepherd who suffered from hip dysplasia and arthritis. He received regular acupuncture treatments, took Chinese herbs and had home-cooked congee for his meals. Though he wasn't expected to live past 11 or 12, Merlin lived to be almost 15 years old.

Recipe for Merlin's Magic Congee

Grains should be thoroughly cooked for animals, as they don't really chew their food well. Congee is a Chinese dish made from rice, meat and vegetables that is slow cooked and easy to digest.

In a crock pot or heavy pot with lid add:

- 5 cups of spring or filtered (not tap) water or free-range chicken broth.
- 1 cup rice
- Several pieces of frozen or fresh organic chicken or turkey.
- 1 cup or more of chopped or frozen veggies such as carrots, celery, sweet potato, yams, parsley, string beans.

Use brown rice during the cold winter months. Use white basmati rice for spring or summer.

Add a small handful of raw tonifying herbs such as astragalus, dang gui, ginseng or codenopsis in the congee.

If cooking in a crock pot, set on low and cook for 4-6 hours. If using a heavy pot on the stove, set the flame or electric burner on the lowest setting, and cook for 4-6 hours.

Cooking With Oats

Here is another recipe with oats, to use on special occasions and holidays. Oats are great for relieving stress and calming a nervous dog.

Nikki's Grateful Oats Recipe for Dogs

Boil two cups water, add one cup of quick cooking rolled oats, remove from heat, cover and passively cook for 45 min. Boil ground turkey or ground chicken about two cups drain and cool.

Steam either green beans, baby carrots or sweet potatoes with a couple cloves of fresh garlic so they are soft, let cool. Add a sprig of parsley for good breath and serve in your favorite holiday dog bowl.

Cinnamon Meatballs for Dogs

Here is a meatball recipe for your dog with warming cinnamon for those dogs affected by cold damp winter days. NOTE: **Please do not add onion to this recipe as onion is toxic for dogs.**

Cinnamon Meatballs for Dogs

- 1/2 pound of free range/organic ground chicken or turkey
- 1/4 cup of shredded carrots (optional)
- 3 tablespoons of fresh or dried parsley (great for dog breath)
- 1 teaspoon of salt

- 1/8 cup of parmesan cheese
- 1 egg
- 1 tablespoon of cinnamon

DO NOT ADD ONION!

Heat oven to 375. Line a large baking sheet with non-stick foil. Combine all the ingredients into a large bowl and mix until blended. Form into meatballs and bake for about 20-25 minutes. Allow to cool before serving to your dog!

Organic Chicken or Turkey Jerky Treats

With the recalls of so many dog treats lately why not be safe and make your own? Here is an easy recipe your dog will love and that will save you money too. Please make sure that your dog is not allergic to chicken or turkey before making a batch.

Ingredients:

- Package of organic free range chicken or turkey breasts
- Cookie Sheet
- Preheat Oven to 185 degrees

Please make sure the chicken or turkey is free range, and preferably organic. Clean the breasts. Slice them carefully into long thin strips.

Place the chicken or turkey strips on a non-stick or greased cookie sheet. Bake the strips for about 3 hours in the oven at 185 degrees. Keeping the temperature low will dry the turkey or chicken at a slower rate making it a chewy treat for your dog. Remove from the oven when the strips seem "jerky" enough for your dog. The drier the strips, the better they will keep, but they are also tougher to eat if your dog has dental problems.

Let cool to room temperature before giving one to Fido. Store in plastic bags or containers.

You can also make chicken, turkey or sweet potato treats using an inexpensive dehydrator. For Yang Deficient dogs, cooking is better. For Yin Deficient dogs, dehydration is better.

7.3   Healthy Treats

Make sure the dog cookies and treats are also free of wheat, corn, soy or animal by-products. Other treats such as carrots, apples (without the seeds), and bananas are fine too. Some dogs love these things while others will turn their nose up.

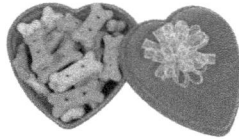

Elk Antler Treats

Elk antlers are a safe and healthy substitute for beef bones or plastic Nymo bones (which contain wheat gluten). No animals are harmed producing these. Every year male elk shed their antlers naturally. In Chinese medicine Elk and Reindeer antlers are used in yang tonic formulas. They are a rich source of nutrients and minerals with no added ingredients.

They also last much longer than a bone. My dog goes through one about every 2 months. She LOVES them. They are also very safe as they do not have splinters, they don't get slimy and they have no odor too. Make sure you buy only the antlers from the USA. You can find these in the better pet stores and on-line. If you buy an antler that is breaking easily or has splinters it is defective, probably too old. (Warning: at least one of the big box Pet food chain stores sells these without checking if they're good.)

7.4   Dog Bowls

Elevate dishes off the floor for older dogs or those suffering from health problems to make it easier for them to reach food and water. Use ceramic, stainless steel or Pyrex bowls only. Plastic bowls breed germs and mold and can retain the smell of cleaning products.

7.5   Water for the dog

Research has shown that drugs and chemicals, chlorine and fluoride, metals like lead and cadmium are in our tap water. Drinking tap water can be dangerous for humans and animals. Taking the time to fill a dog's water bowl with fresh filtered water may help prevent cancer and other diseases.

If you do not have a water filter you can purchase a water filter system (Brita products, for example) at many grocery and department stores.

Also, always make sure that a dog has enough water to drink, especially on hot days. To those who don't think this is important, I challenge them to put on a winter coat and stand outside on a hot day with no water for four hours.

Smart Water®

I recommend this brand of water for older pets and those who may suffer from dehydration. Made by a US bottler called Glaceau, "Smart Water begins as an artesian spring in Northern Connecticut. After the water is distilled,a balance of Magnesium, Potassium, and Calcium is introduced, adding electrolytes." This results in a balanced, known quantity of electrolytes. There are similar products available, but check the ingredient list to be sure that they include distilled water (not purified – they aren't the same thing) with the same list of electrolytes.

Smart Water can be found in most grocery and drug stores.

7.6 Foods to Avoid Giving a Dog

- Chocolate
- Macadamia nuts
- Onions
- Grapes
- Pear pips, the kernels of plums, peaches and apricots, apple core pips (contain cyanogenic glycosides resulting in cyanide poisoning)
- Tylenol is a deadly poison for dogs
- Antifreeze
- Potato peelings and green looking potatoes
- Rhubarb leaves
- Moldy/spoiled foods
- Alcohol
- Yeast dough
- Coffee grounds, beans and tea (caffeine)
- Hops (used in home brewing)
- Tomato leaves and stems (green parts)
- Broccoli (in large amounts)
- Raisins and grapes
- Cigarettes, tobacco, cigars: toxic if they eat it and second hand smoke
- Rawhide- can get stuck in the throat
- Cow's hooves and pig's ears: risk of salmonella

- Milk: dogs do not have the enzymes to digest lactose

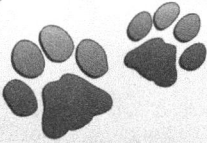

The Native Americas revered the wolf, coyote and the domestic dog.

Chapter 8

Reading list

Recommended Books:

1. *The Nature Of Animal Healing*, Martin Goldstein, DVM

2. *Clinical Handbook of Chinese Veterinary Herbal Medicine*, Signe Beebe, DVM, Michael Salewski, DVM. Lorena Monda, DOM, John Scott, DOM

3. *Four Paws, Five Directions*, Cheryl Schwartz, DVM

4. *K'an Chinese Herbals For Animals*, Steve Marsden, DVM, L.Ac.

5. *Handbook For Veterinarians*, Steve Mardsen

6. *Veterinary Acupuncture*, Alan M Klide VMD, Shui H Kung PH.D

7. *The Good The Bad and The Furry*, Edwin J. Sayres

8. *How To Be Your Dogs Best Friend*, The Monks Of New Skete

9. *The Well Connected Dog*, Amy Snow and Nancy Zidonis

Journals:

1. *Whole Dog Journal*

2. *Bark Magazine*

Chapter 9

Resource Guide

Bach Flower Rescue Remedy & Flower Essences:

Nelsons

21 High Street Ste 302

North Andover MA 01845

www.nelsons.net

www.bachremedies.com

www.rescueremedy.com/pets

Thundershirt:

www.thundershirt.com

866-892-2078

DVDs For Animal Acupuncture Acupressure Point Location:

TallGrass Animal Acupuncture Institute

www.animalacupressure.com

888-841-7211

tallgrass@animalacupressure.com

Relaxing Music for Dogs & Cats

Through a Dogs Ear

www.ThroughADogsEar.com

800-788-0949

NCCAOM approved CEU/PDAs for Veterinary Acupuncture and Books:

Zen Paws Healing

www.zenpawshealing.com

Four Paws Acupuncture

www.fourpawsacupuncture.com

k9acudoc@gmail.com

Bibliography

DVM. Beebe, Signe, DVM. Salewski Micheal, DOM. Monda Lorena, and DOM John Scott. *Clinical Handbook of Chinese Veterinary Herbal Medicine.* Herbal Medicine Press, Placitas, NM, 2006.

Dan Bensky and Randall Barolet. *Chinese Herbal Medicine, Formulas and Strategies.* Eastland Press, Seattle, WA, 1990.

Fiorenzo Fiorone. *The Encyclopedia Of Dogs.* Hart-Davis, Mac Gibbob, London, UK.

Jake Fratkin. *Chinese Classics, Popular Herbal Formulas, Guide for the Practioner.* Shya Publications, Boulder, CO, 1990.

DVM Goldstein, Martin. *The Nature of Animal Healing.* Ballantine Books, New York, NY, 1999.

OMD Kaptchuk, Ted. *The Web That Has No Weaver, Un-*

derstanding Chinese Medicine. Congdon and Weed, Inc., New York, NY, 1989.

Alan VMD Klide and Ph.D. Kung, Shiu. Veterinary Acupuncture. University of Pennsylvania Press, PA, 1977.

Lee-kin. A Handbook of Acupuncture Treatment for Dogs and Cats. Medicine and Health Publishing Co., Hong Kong.

Giovanni Maciocia. The Foundations of Chinese Medicine, A Comprehensive Text for Acupuncturists and Herbalists. Churchill Livingstone, New York, NY, 1989.

Bobbie DVM Mammato. American Red Cross Pet First Aid. Times Mirror Company, Boston MA, 1997.

Gabriel Mojay. Aromatherapy For Healing The Spirit. Henry Holt and Company, New York, NY, 1996.

Monks of New Skete. Divine Canine, The Monk's Way To A Happy Obedient Dog. Hyperion, New York, NY, 2007.

The Monks of New Skete. How To Be Your Dog's Best Friend. Little, Brown and Company, New York, NY, 2002.

The Monks of New Skete. *I & Dog*. Yorkville Press, New York, NY, 2003.

Mechthild Scheffer. *Bach Flowers for Crisis Care, Remedies for Emotional and Psychological Well-being*. Healing Arts Press, Rochester, Vermont, 2006.

DVM Schwartz, Cheryl. *Four Paws, Five Directions, A Guide to Chinese Medicine for Cats and Dogs*. Celestial Arts, Berkeley, CA, 1996.

Amy Snow and Nancy Zidonis. *The Well Connected Dog, A Guide to Canine Acupressure*. Tallgrass Publishers, Larkspur, CO, 1999.

Sam Stall. *The Good, The Bad and the Furry, Choosing The Dog That's Right For You*. Quirk Books, Philadelphia, PA, 2005.

Cheng Xingnong. *Chinese Acupuncture and Moxabustion*. Foreign Languages Press, Beijing, China, 1987.

Martin Zucker. *The Veterinarian's Guide to Natural Remedies for Dogs*. Three Raven Press, New York NY, 1999.

Index

About the Author

Jeanie Mossa Kraft is an acupuncturist and Chinese herbalist and owner of Four Paws Acupuncture and Zen Paws Healing. She earned a Master of Traditional Oriental Medicine degree from Pacific College of Oriental Medicine at San Diego, California, and taught at the Canadian College of Oriental Medicine in Toronto, Canada. She has been treating dogs (and humans) with acupuncture since 1995. She has previously worked as a steel worker, a glass artist and dog walker. She lives in Alexandria, Virginia with her husband and a menagerie of animals.

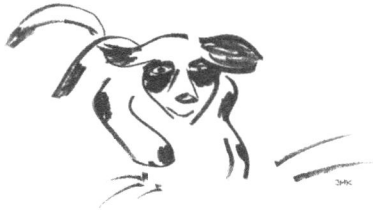

She speaks fluent canine.

About the Coauthor

Norman Kraft is an acupuncturist, herbalist, and author. He earned a Master of Traditional Oriental Medicine degree from the Pacific College of Oriental Medicine at San Diego, California. He is the former Dean of the Canadian College of Oriental Medicine and taught at the Pacific College of Oriental Medicine at New York. He has completed additional graduate studies in counseling and clinical hypnotherapy. Mr. Kraft has been practicing Chinese medicine since 1980. He lives in Alexandria, VA with his wife Jeanie and a growing collection of animals.

He does not treat dogs, has not been a dog walker and does not speak fluent canine. He's the left brain of the family.

Contact Us

For more information about canine acupuncture, including PDA courses for acupuncturists, visit our websites below.

Four Paws Acupuncture: www.fourpawsacupuncture.com

Zen Paws Healing: www.zenpawshealing.com